# Doctor, Is Liposuction Right for Me?

# Doctor, Is Liposuction Right for Me?

*Baldev S Sandhu M.D.*

Writers Club Press

San Jose New York Lincoln Shanghai

# Doctor, Is Liposuction Right for Me?

Writers Club Press
an imprint of iUniverse.com, Inc.

For information address:
iUniverse.com, Inc.
5220 S 16th, Ste. 200
Lincoln, NE 68512
www.iuniverse.com

ISBN: 0-595-19124-X

Printed in the United States of America

*To my darling wife, Lilly, and my loving children, Raji and Sasha.*

*For all the love and support you have given me.*

# Contents

# List of Illustrations

# Foreword

This book is meant to be read as a general introduction to what lipo-suction can and cannot achieve. After reading it you will be a much more informed patient and it has been my experience that informed patients, who have realistic expectations and goals from their pro-posed cosmetic surgery, are more satisfied with their surgery and have better rapport with their surgeon.

However, a book is not a substitute for a consultation with a plastic surgeon who can actually examine you and discuss your specific prob-lems with you after having the benefit of actually seeing and touching the problem areas. My belief, however, is that you will be better pre-pared after reading this book to ask the questions that are important to you during your consultation.

A thorough consultation in combination with the knowledge gained from this book will put you well onto the road to answering the question: Is Liposuction right for Me? I am always interested in hear-ing about this surgery from a patient's perspective and your feedback, either before or after you have surgery is always welcome. You can reach me easily by e-mailing me at sandhuplas@aol.com. I can't prom-ise to respond to each e-mail individually but let me take this opportu-nity to thank you in advance if you choose to do so. You never know I may be able to incorporate your experiences and insights in future edi-tions of this book!

# Acknowledgements

I would like to thank all my patients, who have honored me by selecting my artistic and surgical skills to help them achieve their goals of improving their appearance via plastic surgery.

I am even more indebted to all the patients who have agreed to allow me to use their pictures in this book, but I have changed all these patient's names in the pictures and anecdotes to preserve their privacy.

Every physician owes a debt of gratitude to all those who taught him or her, and here I would like to thank the many fine physicians and surgeons who have guided me throughout my career. In particular I would like to mention Alan Shons M.D., James Lehman M.D., Bahman Guyuron, M.D., Kelman Cohen M.D. and Austin Mehrhoff M.D.

In writing this book I relied heavily on my daughter, Raji, for her editorial guidance although I freely accept responsibility for any literary shortcomings in my writing. I am also grateful to Santokh Lalli and Chris Cordes for their computer skills in typesetting and converting my photographs to electronic files ready for publishing in this digital age.

# Chapter 1

## Thinking about Liposuction?

Liposuction is the most common procedure performed by plastic surgeons in America today. The American Society of Plastic Surgeons in a survey of its members found that they had performed 229,588 liposuction procedures in the year 2000 alone! So, if you are contemplating liposuction, the statistics show that you are not alone in doing so.

One American in every thousand underwent this procedure last year by a Board Certified plastic surgeon and this probably vastly underestimates the reality of the situation because the American Society of Plastic Surgeon's survey does not include dermatologists, ENT's, and other assorted physicians who offer this procedure to their patients. I doubt if there is anyone who has not looked at his or her figure in the mirror and thought, "If only I could get rid of this roll of fat!" and wondered about the possibilities of liposuction.

This book is for everyone who has had precisely that thought. The purpose of this book is to answer your questions, as fully and frankly as possible, about this procedure which has so many myths and misconceptions surrounding it. This book describes what liposuction can achieve and what it cannot achieve, so that, if after reading this book, you do decide to go ahead and have liposuction you will have a realistic understanding of what to expect from initial consultation through final recovery.

This book is written from the patient's perspective. It assumes no prior medical knowledge, and takes you through the steps of waking up one day, looking in the mirror, and deciding, that if everyone else is achieving a better body through liposuction then maybe you should look into it as well. Almost certainly some of your best friends have had liposuction, and just as certainly a high proportion of them will lie brazenly to you and deny any such thing. This is where "Doctor, Is Liposuction Right for Me?" comes in. I hope it answers your questions in a forthright manner and will help you decide if you want to take that first initial step of seeking a consultation with a qualified plastic surgeon and how to go about finding one that best suits your needs.

Liposuction is a purely elective procedure and you have the luxury of time to investigate and decide if this surgery is for you. Make no mistake about it though, liposuction is surgery and should only be performed by a qualified surgeon so it is important to do your research, not just on the procedure itself, but the surgeon you ultimately select to perform this procedure for you. Like any surgical procedure liposuction carries risks and benefits but, unlike many surgeries that have to be performed on an emergency basis, the patient considering liposuction has the luxury of time to investigate the pros and cons of this surgery.

Thus, the most important differentiating feature of liposuction, like that of all cosmetic procedures, from other "necessary" surgeries is that you have the luxury of taking time to make your decision to go ahead and have the surgery and researching your decision thoroughly, because, after all, it is you, the patient, who is making the decision as to wether you *need* liposuction and want to go ahead with the surgery.

Nevertheless patients are always asking me "Doctor, Do I need liposuction?" The answer to that question is always the same: "Unless you are an actor or model that depend for your living on your physical appearance, there is no-one who must have liposuction. You can live the rest of your life quite easily without this surgery"

When I answer this way the patient usually replies, "I knew that!" with a look on their face as if to say, "What kind of fool do you think I am Doctor?" At this point I usually smile and say, "What you really mean is: in my case, will the cost and risk of liposuction be worth the benefits?"

That is the question this book is designed to help you answer for yourself, because every patient has to make up their own mind about this question, for themselves. And let me add, sometimes the answer the patient comes up with does not meet the approval of their spouse or other loved ones. I have seen instances where a man wanted to have liposuction and his wife was dead set against it and, just as inappropriate, a boyfriend pushing his girlfriend to have liposuction when she obviously did not want to. Managing and discussing such psychodramas are well outside the scope of this book although obviously they impact on the patient's "need" for the surgery. This book simply points out the realities of what liposuction can and cannot achieve and leaves the decisions up to you.

Reading this book at home you will have the luxury of time to digest the information presented and you will be able to write down any questions that apply to your particular situation so you will be well prepared when you go for consultation with a plastic surgeon to ask the questions that are important to you to make an informed decision as to wether liposuction is right for you. To help you in doing so, at the back of this book, there are some questions, which you might want to have answered during your consultation, and there you can write down any additional questions that you come up with also.

# Chapter 2

## The history of Liposuction

Liposuction is a young procedure and was introduced in the United States only in the early 1980's from France where it had been developed by a French surgeon, Yves-Gerard Ilouz, who is commonly credited as the father of liposuction. The development of surgical procedures tends to be evolutionary rather than revolutionary but the publication of *"Une nouvelle technique pour les lypodystrophies localisees"* in France by Dr Ilouz marked the beginning of a remarkable change in surgical thinking. He did not have an easy time at first convincing surgeons that the procedure he first reported in 1980 was a significant addition to the compendium of cosmetic surgery procedures because previous attempts by plastic surgeons to shave out fat from underneath the skin through small incisions had resulted in very high complication rates.

The procedure Dr Ilouz described was done under general anesthesia, with the instrumentation available at that time. Through small incisions fat was literally scraped out by an instrument referred to as a curette, which was attached via tubing to a high vacuum pump which allowed the fat to be suctioned out of the body. Dr Ilouz used a *blunt* tipped curette, which caused less injury than the *sharp* scraping instruments used by prior surgeons and relied on the high negative pressure of the suction vacuum to pull the fat out of the body.

While the results were dramatic, the complication rates were still significant and included haematomas, blood loss, severe bruising and occasional skin loss. Despite these problems it was clear that Ilouz was onto something and that, contrary to prior surgical thinking, removal

4

of significant amounts of subcutaneous fat through small incision was, in fact, possible. The search was on, almost immediately, to make this procedure safer and many surgeons around the world have contributed to the development of the technique that rapidly came to be known as liposuction.

What had been revolutionary was the demonstration that fat could be removed with relative safety through tiny incisions. Since then there have been many evolutionary steps, both in the instrumentation and the surgical technique, to try and make the procedure simpler and safer and many plastic surgeons have contributed to the evolution of the procedure to make liposuction into one of the most commonly performed surgeries in the United States today.

The first modification of the technique was to try and reduce the blood loss during liposuction and to this end surgeons started injecting the areas to be worked on with a dilute mixture of adrenaline, (to constrict the local blood vessels and thereby minimize bleeding), and local anesthetic to provide post-operative pain relief. This was referred to as the "wet technique" to differentiate it from liposuction as originally described by Ilouz which was referred to as the "dry technique".

Early on it became clear that this "wet technique" significantly reduced the complication rate particularly with respect to the incidence of bleeding, haematomas and associated skin damage or loss. A further advantage was that since the operative sites were numb from the local anesthetic it was not necessary to put the patient under general anesthesia and liposuction could be carried out under light sedation.

Well, if pre-treatment with a little local anesthesia and adrenaline was good then maybe using a lot of this mixture, the injectate, would be better and this gave rise to the "super-wet technique" in which the amount of fluid injected was equal to the amount of fat to be removed. Thus, if the surgeon estimated he was going to remove one and a half litres of fat, in the super-wet technique, he would pre-inject with one and a half liters of injectate for a ratio of one-to-one of injectate to fat being extracted.

Originally, you have to remember, the amount of fat being removed was relatively small, simply to sculpture the body and change the body's shape in young healthy patients—a procedure that I refer to as *finesse liposuction*. I use the term finesse liposuction for those patients in whom I am trying to simply sculpture an already beautiful patient who is near, or even below, their ideal weight and really don't require a lot of fat to be removed. In the patient requiring finesse liposuction the superwet technique causes too much swelling and distortion of the affected area, as you really want to see the changes in shape as they are occurring during the surgery.

These patients seeking finesse liposuction are completely different from those patients who are ten per cent or more above their ideal body weight, and are more concerned with what I classify as *liposuction for volume reduction*. Although both these classes of patients are having liposuction, they really are undergoing completely different surgeries in terms of the physiological changes that the body undergoes during and after the surgery and in terms of the recovery time involved.

The next development in liposuction, *the tumescent technique*, is applicable only to those patients undergoing liposuction for volume reduction. In the tumescent technique large volumes of fluid are used to pre-inject the operative site and is therefore not applicable to those patients in whom finesse is important. The tumescent technique is involved in large volume liposuction where up to five liters of fat are to be removed in a single surgical session. Here the operative site is distended with two to three times the volume of the fat expected to be removed causing the operative site to become firm, or in medical terminology, tumescent. Thus, if a liposuction of five liters is planned, then the area is injected with ten or more liters of the tumescent fluid. Now wether volume liposuction is a good idea or not is a totally separate question that we cover in the chapter on volume liposuction. The only point I want to make here is that finesse liposuction and volume liposuction are completely different procedures and a lot of confusion arises from not accurately separating these two procedures into different categories. The risks associated with volume liposuction include all those associated with finesse liposuction plus other significant risks attributable to the large volume fluid shifts involved in liposuction for volume and we will cover these risks in the chapter specifically devoted to the risks of liposuction surgery.

Other developments in liposuction techniques since the development of the original method are related to improved instrumentation. Of these the most important has been the development of ultrasonic probes that deliver fat liquefying ultrasonic energy to the fat and allow the fat to be then extracted with less force than if the fat had not been "melted" prior to suctioning it out. The ability to deliver this fat melting energy directly to the area to be treated is a significant advance because in some areas of the body the fat globules are tightly bound amongst themselves and to the adjacent fibrous tissue and are difficult to extract with traditional liposuction. While *ultrasonic liposuction* represents a significant advance in being able to perform liposuction the additional energy delivered by the ultrasound probe also carries additional risks. The positives and negatives of ultrasonic liposuction are addressed in the chapter on risks of liposuction. Suffice it here to say that ultrasonic liposuction has enabled the treatment of areas that responded poorly to traditional liposuction such as fat in the male breast or fat in the buttocks.

The most recent evolution of liposuction techniques is "power liposuction". To understand this, remember that in the traditional liposuction technique the liposuction cannula is moved by the surgeon's arm in the subcutaneous space and as the liposuction cannula travels through the subcutaneous fat, this fat is drawn into the cannula and then pulled into the suction tubing by the vacuum pump attached to the end of it.

In *"power liposuction"* the surgeon introduces the cannula into the area to be liposuctioned and then the cannula is moved back and forth by electromechanical power delivered to the cannulae by a small electrical motor or similar device.

Thus, the energy that was being generated by the surgeon's arm, to move the cannula through the subcutaneous fat, has been replaced by this outside source of power. Clearly, this could be a significant benefit for the *surgeon*. There are reported cases of surgeon's suffering from repetitive stress injury of the arm and elbow due to the repetitive to and fro motion involved in performing liposuction which gives rise to the disabling condition commonly referred to as "tennis elbow". Avoidance of this problem for the surgeon seems to be the main potential benefit of the so-called "power liposuction" – as I have been unable to see any improvement in the clinical results achieved using these electro-mechanical devices.

Another difference in techniques is the means of applying vacuum suction to the cannula. Most surgeons utilize a high power pump attached by clear tubing to the cannula to generate the negative pressure required to suction the fat out of the patient's body. Negative pressure can also be achieved by simply using a syringe attached to the cannula and this is highly effective also and the choice of some surgeons but most surgeons prefer to use a vacuum pump for technical ease in performing the operation.

Like any surgical technique liposuction will continue to evolve and be refined over the years so if there is anything that you read or hear about that I have not covered write it down at the end of chapter 13 "Things you might want to discuss with your Surgeon" so that you can get the most up to date and detailed information when you go for consultation.

# Chapter 3

## Does Liposuction really work?

This is the most common question asked by patients—bar none. For some incredulous patients it almost seems like a dream come true. Just imagine being able to get rid of those unsightly fat deposits in one short surgical session!! Other patients are more skeptical and have heard stories about people who had liposuction where it worked for a while, only for the patient to subsequently put the weight back on again. The myths and misconceptions about liposuction that patients have reported to me during consultation are legend, but the most common one is that liposuction does not "work".

Let me put it in no uncertain terms. Liposuction works! There is no more direct and dramatic attack on those unsightly bulges of fat than directly removing them with liposuction.

For the patient seeking finesse liposuction there is simply no other means to achieve the desired results. These are the patients who are at or near their ideal body weight and are simply disproportionate. Look at our first patient, Andrea (Figs 6.1-4), in the finesse liposuction chapter. Her problem is typical of the patient who is an ideal candidate for liposuction. Her thighs are too wide for the size of her waist, breasts and shoulders. Despite being extremely attractive and at the ideal weight for her height when she goes shopping for clothes, she has to buy pants a size larger than her top to accommodate her thighs. If you listen carefully to this patient she will tell you a very typical story. When she puts on weight it seems to go directly to her thighs and when, by dint of diet and exercise, she drops that weight she loses it, not from her thighs, but her face or her breasts or some other place she can't afford to lose the fat.

After a few cycles of weight gain and loss her hips are actually bigger than when she started! In such a patient her high affinity fat receptors are located in her outer thighs. When there is fat available in the bloodstream these high affinity fat cell receptors grab onto the fat first and when Andrea loses weight these are the fat cells that are last to let go of the fat. This concept of *high affinity fat receptors* explains why in each patient seeking finesse liposuction, the unsightly fat seems to congregate in one particular spot and the patients cannot get rid of it by diet or exercise.

In patient Elizabeth (Fig. 6.13), these high affinity fat receptors are in the neck and in Bernadette (Fig. 7.1) these high affinity receptors are in the back. In each of these patients even with rigorous dieting and weight loss these unwanted fat deposits are not going to go away. In fact, quite the reverse, when the patient puts on any weight it is going straight to these high affinity sites and makes them look even bigger!

The common misconception is that you can exercise these unsightly fat deposits away. In these patients it is simply not true. No matter how many lateral leg lifts Andrea (Fig. 6.1-6.4) performs she will build up those muscles but that will have no direct effect on the fat overlying that muscle. Just as exercising the lateral leg muscles will not reduce the fat overlying them exercising the pectoral or chest muscle will not cause an increase or decrease in the size of the breasts. These are two sides of the same coin: exercising a particular muscle group has no effect on the fat or tissue overlying that muscle. Exercise can increase the size of muscles, of course, and is an important part of any weight reduction regimen but the concept of "spot reduction" of fat through exercising the affected part is a total myth.

Patient Bernadette could never spot reduce away the fat under her chin even though her jaw muscles are in continuous use while talking, speaking and chewing during the day. In patients with disproportion there is essentially no other way to correct that disproportion than by surgically removing those high affinity fat cells, that cause the dispro-portion, with liposuction.

If disproportion is your problem, I can tell you confidently that noth-ing else will work to correct your disproportion. Liposuction is the only available method to correct this disproportion. The term liposculpture is sometimes used to signify this correction of disproportion, but, of course, this is simply liposuction under a different name.

Having liposuction does not mean you can abandon diet, exercise and weight control. The inescapable truth of the matter is that if you take in more calories than you use on a daily basis some of those calo-ries will be stored in your body, *as fat*, for future use. However, even when patients do gain weight, after liposuction, for finesse, it is unlikely to go back to those areas that bothered the patient. The reason for this is that those high affinity receptors are simply no longer there screaming out for the fat to congregate in that area.

The importance of diet, weight control and exercise are even more important in the patient considering what I refer to as liposuction for volume reduction. These patients are generally more than 15% over-weight and while they may be disproportionate in how this excess weight is distributed the performance of liposuction is primarily for volume reduction, which will clearly reduce their size and allow them to fit into their clothes better and look better. However, in these patients the importance of diet and exercise post-operatively cannot be overemphasized!

In fact, in some of these patients rigorous diet and exercise will allow them to reduce their size significantly and this gives rise to the most important question that these patients ask: Should I postpone or perhaps even forego liposuction altogether in favor of diet and exer-cise? My answer to this question is always as follows: If you have tried your level best to lose the excess fat through diet and exercise then we can perform liposuction to help you along the way. If you haven't already tried your very level best to lose the excess fat through diet and exercise then you should go on a twelve-week trial of a rigorous diet and exercise program before you even consider liposuction. The next question from the patient is always then what do you recommend in terms of an exercise and diet program?

This question deserves a book of its own and having been asked this question so often I have written "The Plastic Surgeon's Diet Book" which I recommend to my patients and hope to have in bookstores soon.

This is not to diminish the role of volume liposuction. It is a tremendously successful procedure. If you remove four liters of fat through liposuction, that is 4000 grams of fat gone, and since each gram of fat equals 9.3 calories then in one surgical session you can remove the equivalent of 37200 calories. To put that in context if you were to go on a restricted 1200 calorie a day diet as opposed to a normal 1800 calorie diet it would take 62 days of sticking to this rigorous diet to achieve the same loss of fat. In reality this is a tremendously difficult thing to do and most of my patients are like Jaclyn (Figs. 7.15-20), illustrated in the chapter on volume liposuction, who decide that to achieve the body they want they need not only to manage their diet and exercise but also utilize liposuction to help them to their goal of a new and improved body. These patients, however, have to accept that to maintain their new bodyshape they have to be much more aware about their diet and exercise than those patients who had liposuction for finesse simply because they are prone to putting on weight in the first place.

The answer, therefore, is, yes liposuction does work, but it is not a cure-all. It is, simply put, a two-hour procedure during which the surgeon gets one chance to change the shape of your body. It is not a passport to go to McDonald's and especially for those patients who are considering liposuction for volume reduction they have to be aware that it was their diet and exercise program, or lack thereof, that got them into that situation where they were considering liposuction in the first place. If they don't change their lifestyle and eating habits they may well end up being one of those patients who end up saying, "Well I had liposuction and it didn't do any good!"

Realistic expectations and an understanding of what liposuction can and cannot do for you is the key to a successful result and a happy patient. After all, in cosmetic surgery, the only measure of a successful outcome is if the patient is happy and satisfied with the result. The problem for the surgeon is to try and gauge wether the patient has realistic expectations or not of the proposed procedure. In the next chapter, let me tell you about some of the experiences I have had which illustrate this problem for the surgeon.

# Chapter 4

## Will I be happy with the Surgery?

There is only one good reason why patients should have cosmetic surgery: to make themselves happy! The decision to undergo surgery is not made lightly by any patient but at the core of it all is the patient's understanding that if they look better the world will respond to them in a more positive way, both in social situations and in a business context. The expectation of a positive psychic payback is the reason why patients invest in cosmetic surgery and I believe this increase in self-esteem, as well as their new body is what patients are really achieving from any cosmetic surgery, including liposuction. After all, if the world treated unattractive people and beautiful people the same, why would anyone bother to try to look attractive? Patients understand this intuitively.

Those patients who are unhappy after surgery, in some way, have not had those expectations satisfied. Let me illustrate this by a patient I saw in consultation recently. This patient had liposuction a few years earlier by another well-known plastic surgeon in New York City, where I practice. The patient was clearly dissatisfied with the result and was blaming this surgeon for her dissatisfaction. I knew the surgeon personally and knew him to be an excellent, board-certified plastic surgeon. However, even if I hadn't, I would simply tell the patient the truth, which is, "I don't know what you looked like two years ago before the surgery or what you looked like after the surgery, so I really can't comment on that, or explain why you are dissatisfied. Let's talk about what I see today and what I think I can do for you"

"Yes", said the patient, "but will I be satisfied with your surgery, and what happens if I'm not satisfied". The answer to this question of course is that there is no guarantee that a patient will be satisfied because satisfaction is purely in the patient's psyche. Also if the previous surgeon couldn't satisfy the patient what was to make me think that I could? Of course I declined to operate on this patient, but even in my own practice with my own patients it's difficult to tell who will be happy and who will not.

I had a patient named Bruce that, when I saw him initially in consultation, I was not really sure wether he was a good candidate for liposuction. First of all he was a big guy, about six feet two, and weighed almost 220lbs so he was significantly overweight. I was not really sure that liposuction of four liters, the maximum that I will remove in one surgical sitting, really would make a significant difference to him. I told him quite frankly that I wasn't sure that liposuction would really make that much difference to him and that maybe he should lose some weight prior to considering liposuction. Bruce, however, really wanted to have the surgery, and in fact had vacation time coming in two weeks from his job as a computer programmer and that was when he wanted to have the surgery. He promised me that he would go on a diet and exercise program and that the liposuction would help motivate him to do so and stick with it.

After discussing the pros and cons, we went ahead and did the surgery. Everything went well and when I saw Bruce in follow-up he looked significantly better but still no physique that would turn the ladies' heads. Bruce, however, was ecstatic with the results. Though I was happy about that, I was also curious as to why he was so happy.

Then he told me the truth, "Well, Doctor, I was able to give up my job as a computer programmer because I got a walk–on part on one of the day time soap operas". Knowing what computer programmers get paid and what the Equity minimum that the soap opera was probably paying I didn't think of that as a move-up, at least financially. Furthermore, I was pretty convinced in my own mind that the liposuction had nothing to do with Bruce landing the acting job and told him so. It didn't matter! Bruce was convinced that the liposuction had given him the confidence to land that job and he didn't mind that he had traded in a high paying job as a computer programmer for a low paying acting job. In fact he was not concerned about the money at all, but thrilled, as he put it "To give up toiling at my vocation of computer programming for the joy of being able to pursue my avocation of act-ing—and I really think the liposuction helped me to get there". I was happy for him and also happy to take the credit. But the opposite can also happen.

Jane had just come to New York to pursue a modeling career. She was, I can report quite objectively, as someone who spends most of my time looking at the human form, just gorgeous. Undoubtedly a ten! When she came in for consultation she had just the teeniest amount of excess fat around the bikini line and she also wanted a small hump on her nose taken care of. She was a great candidate for both surgeries and the rhinoplasty and liposuction went beautifully with a really fan-tastic result, but when she came into the office post-operatively she was depressed.

I pointed out that the surgical result was quite excellent. "Yes, I know," she said "But I still have the same lousy apartment, I haven't landed any of the modeling assignments I've been up for, and my boyfriend and I just broke up. Maybe I just shouldn't have had the sur-gery". It's difficult for the surgeon when the patient is unhappy fol-lowing a successful surgical result. I could only imagine what her state of mind would have been if she had developed an infection or some other complication following surgery!

This brings me to the next question which prospective patients have to confront. What are the risks of surgery and are they prepared to handle them? Liposuction like all cosmetic surgery is a choice that the patient has made with the hopes and aim of improving their appear-ance. If for any reason, those goals or other expectations that they had in the back of their mind, are not met the patient will naturally be as disappointed as Jane was.

But what if the patient has a problem such as a wound infection, blood clot, an adverse anesthetic event or other serious problem during or after surgery? Often these patients will go into a profound depression. Not only have their goals of an improved appearance not been met, but also they have the problem of requiring additional time off work, additional expenses for taking care of the problems and may even require additional surgery. On top of all this, their friends and family, who may not have been told of the proposed surgery, are rarely supportive in such a situation leaving the patient even more depressed and isolated. Thus, while liposuction is extremely safe and complications are rare, the patient has to understand that if _they_ are the patient who suffers a complication they really will not care about the other ninety-nine percent whose surgery was complication free and are pleased with the results of their surgery.

For that one patient the complication rate is 100% and while no one likes to think about unhappy thoughts, part of the preparation for surgery is to consider if you really could handle such a problem if it occurred. Read the next chapter carefully and while all the complications outlined have an extremely low probability if you think that you could not handle such a problem emotionally and financially then perhaps cosmetic surgery is not for you.

Let me just illustrate for you the kind of thing, while rare, is the type of problem patients don't like to think about. I performed abdominal liposuction, not a finesse liposuction but one for volume reduction, on a thirty-year-old teacher during spring break. I removed four liters of fat, using the tumescent technique, and the surgery was uneventful. Four days later she called me saying that her left leg was swollen. I asked her to come into the office and after examining her it was clear to me that, most likely, she had developed a blood clot in her leg, technically referred to as a deep vein thrombosis. Now this can happen after any surgery, anywhere in the body (because of changes in the blood clotting system in response to surgery), although it is a relatively rare complication.

The patient was distraught when I told her my diagnosis and even more so when I told her that she would have to be admitted to the hospital to have some tests to confirm the diagnosis. Now this complication needs to be treated aggressively because a piece of the blood clot in the leg can break off and travel to the lung causing a pulmonary embolus, which can be potentially fatal. After hearing this, the patient agreed to be hospitalized and the tests confirmed my diagnosis. A hematologist was consulted and the patient was commenced on intravenous blood thinners and then slowly transferred to oral blood thinners and was discharged from the hospital after five days. Nevertheless she had to stay on the blood thinners for months and visit the hematologist regularly during that time to have her blood checked.

Needless to say the patient was extremely upset! Firstly, she was not able to return to her teaching position on a timely basis after spring break because she was hospitalized. Secondly, she had the cost of hospitalization and the physician fees from her hematologist, and all those blood tests. Fortunately, most of these costs were covered by her health insurance but then she still had the time factor involved in visiting the hematologist's office weekly following her discharge from hospital.

Even while this patient did not have any permanent problems, and in fact had a nice result from the surgery, like any normal human being she did suffer from remorse that she had put herself through all this, as she said, "just for vanity". Now while such problems are rare, and liposuction when performed by a surgeon certified by the American Board of Plastic Surgery is an extremely safe procedure, the possibility of problems remains and if you are the unlucky patient who draws the short straw for you that problem is a hundred percent. If you are the kind of person uncomfortable with any level of risk then liposuction might not be for you. Patients understandably want to be assured that everything is going to go well with their surgery but no surgeon can give such an assurance. In the next chapter we will take a closer look at the risks of liposuction surgery.

# Chapter 5

## Risks of Liposuction

Liposuction, like any surgical procedure, carries some risks and while no patient likes to think negatively it is important to discuss the risks involved with liposuction as for any other surgery. Just because it is cosmetic or "beauty" surgery does not mean the risks are any less than any other comparable surgical procedure such as hernia repair or cholecystectomy.

When I talk to patients I remind them that deaths have been reported following liposuction just as they have been with other surgical procedures, which are thought to be low or moderate risk. Although the probability of death, related to liposuction, is of the order of about one in fifty thousand it is an inevitable fact that surgery, by its very nature, carries risks and for some patients even this extremely low probability will dissuade them from having surgery. That is good and well, and as it should be.

In the broadest of possible terms the other risks of liposuction are related to anesthetic risk, infection and bleeding, all of which can happen with any surgery.

### Anasthetic Risk

Having a well trained anesthesiologist in attendance, even when the surgery is done under local anesthesia, can minimize anesthetic risk. There remains a great deal of confusion amongst the general public about each of the terms used regarding anesthesia so let me describe how I prefer to perform liposuction. The patient has an IV started and running and their vital signs, EKG and oxygen levels are monitored. The patient is then given a short acting Valium-type drug called Versed, (technically classified as a hypnotic agent) and this enables me to inject the areas to be operated on with the local anesthetic fluid. In finesse liposuction, I inject only enough to anaesthetize the area and not to distort the tissue. In liposuction for volume, I inject a more dilute anesthetic solution but in much larger volumes. I then wait ten to fifteen minutes to allow the local anesthetic agent to work and for the patient to fully recover from the effect of the Versed. I can then perform the liposuction with the patient awake and able to move around, which of course is a great help in cases where I am working on multiple areas of the patients' body. I have tried injecting the local anesthetic fluid without the benefit of Versed or a similar agent, but have found that few patients can tolerate this with equanimity. The benefit of giving the patients Versed is that the local anesthetic agent can be injected without the patient feeling it and by the time the Versed has worn off the operative sites are totally numb and ready to be operated on.

The important thing for the patient to understand is that local anesthetics selectively desensitize only the nerve fibers that carry pain. The nerve fibers that carry feelings for hot and cold, touch and vibration are unaffected, so that you will feel the surgeon's hands touching you, but you will feel no pain. Patients understand, intellectually, that this is the safest way to perform liposuction, but many patients are uncomfortable with the idea of watching someone work on them. These patients are more comfortable being sedated throughout the procedure, which means that they are given sufficient anesthesia so that they don't know what is going on, but at all times, they are breathing by themselves without any artificial support for their breathing. This is often referred to as sedation anesthesia or "twilight anesthesia" from the fact that it resembles being in a very deep sleep and is very different from general anesthesia where the patient *cannot* breath for themselves and require a breathing tube attached to a ventilator to breathe for them. This often requires the patient's muscles to be paralyzed so they cannot move and of course requires reversal of the anesthetic agents before the breathing tube can be removed.

Now, while my preference is to perform the procedure essentially under local anesthesia because of what I believe to be the lower risks associated with it, if patients prefer sedation anesthesia or general anesthesia that is fine too. In fact many surgeons only perform lipo-suction under general anesthesia because they feel more comfortable knowing that the patient's airway is already intubated and under con-trol, and feel that the additional medications required to achieve this are worth the risk.

Most plastic surgeons will discuss their preferred anesthetic tech-nique with you and why that is their preference at the time of your con-sultation. However, if you prefer an alternate technique you should discuss that with the anesthesiologist and surgeon prior to the surgery.

## Infection

Infections following liposuction are extremely rare and are mini-mized by commencing the patient on antibiotics prior to surgery, so that they have an adequate level of antibiotics on board before the sur-gery and continuing the antibiotics for twenty-four hours after the sur-gery. When infections do occur they are usually trivial and can be treated with local wound care. However, quite rarely, life threatening systemic or body wide infections have been reported with particularly virulent bacteria requiring hospitalization and intensive care.

## Bleeding Problems

As with any surgery, bleeding problems are possible and can result in blood loss if the patient bleeds too much or the blood fails to clot. Excessive clotting of the blood can also be a problem resulting in thrombosis. Either of these problems can give rise to pressure on the overlying skin with damage to the skin including skin loss. The risk of blood loss has shown to be reduced with the superwet or tumescent technique, particularly in high volume liposuctions. Seromas, while rare and technically not bleeding problems need to be mentioned here also. They are collections of straw colored fluid that develop under the skin in the post-operative period. While not serious problems they may require to be drained multiple times before resolution.

## Injury to skin or internal organs

The liposuction cannula can perforate the skin or enter the chest cavity or abdomen and cause damage to internal organs or blood vessels. This results in complications, which are potentially life threatening if not diagnosed quickly and treated aggressively. This risk can be minimized by operating under local anesthesia so that if the cannula enters an area that is not anaesthetized the patient will be able to tell the surgeon right away, whereas if the patient is in "twilight anesthesia" or under general anesthesia detection of vital organ injury may be delayed. Ultrasonic liposuction cannulae, because of the high energy they generate may result in an increased incidence of injury to the skin or internal organs.

## Special risks associated with high volume liposuction

Liposuction is a surgical attack on the body. The larger the volume of fat to be removed the greater the injury to the body. In this book I have separated what I call finesse liposuction, the purpose of which is really to sculpture the patient's shape by removing small amounts of fat, from liposuction for volume reduction, which is defined in my practice as removal of more than 1.5 liters of fat.

The body's response to the surgical trauma of high volume liposuction is best explained to the patient by asking the simple question: "How sick would you expect to be if four liters, or 8.8 pounds, of your body were surgically amputated?" When you put it in those stark terms to patients, they really begin to understand the magnitude of the operation and the care required to manage that level of injury to the body. The care required is of a much greater order of magnitude than liposuction for finesse.

In volume liposuction the fluid shifts generated in the body are great and approach those involved in major crush injuries or other trauma such as a car accident. The patient needs to have their fluid levels managed with same level of care that such an accident victim would receive. They need sufficient fluids to keep the body systems, especially the kidneys, from going into shutdown, but not so much fluid that it will overload the heart and trip the patient into heart failure. This fluid management requires a well-trained surgeon to adequately manage these fluid replacements and while most high volume liposuctions are uneventful clearly they carry a higher level of risk than finesse liposuction. Most of the problems associated with liposuction surgery are attributable to high volume liposuction surgery. By definition, these patients are overweight, which by itself, as an independent scoring factor, will increase the risk for any surgical procedure. In addition, they are having surgery, which puts a greater stress on their body systems than liposuction for finesse. Those body systems, such as the heart and lung, may not be as capable of handling this greater stress because patients who are overweight are unlikely to be as fit as those who are at their ideal weight.

This has been one of the longest chapters in the book, but it pays careful reading and perhaps even re-reading because I believe that no patient should undertake cosmetic surgery without the understanding that this is still surgery and carries real risks. Complication rates *are* extremely low in the modern day practice of liposuction, but they can occur in the best of hands, including my own. As my old chief of surgery said "the only surgeon who doesn't have complications is the surgeon who doesn't operate."

After the actual decision to undergo an elective procedure like liposuction, the next most important choice is choosing a surgeon with the experience to minimize the risks and the ability to manage any complications should they arise. Chapter eleven is dedicated to helping you make this decision.

# Chapter 6

## Finesse Liposuction

In discussing liposuction with my patients I have found it helpful, after examining them, to separate them into the categories of what I call liposuction for finesse, where the goal is simply to make the body more shapely and attractive and volume liposuction where the goal is, literally, to reduce the volume of the patient. In this chapter we will discuss finesse liposuction which generally entails removing no more than 1.5 liters of fat.

These patients, as you will see in the pictures on the following pages, are generally at or near their ideal weight and their problem is simply one of *disproportion*. This problem of disproportion cannot be solved by diet or exercise no matter how much these patients diet or exercise. In fact by the time these patients come to see a plastic surgeon, like myself, they are generally quite frustrated. They had bought into the idea that by diet and exercise they could attain the body they were seeking. Instead, what these patients found was that with a more strenuous exercise regimen and diet program they lost weight from areas they didn't want to lose it and when they put on weight it seemed to zone in to those areas they were trying to lose the fat from.

For this there is a simple explanation. *Not all fat cells are the same.* Some fat cells have a much higher affinity for fat than their neighboring cells. These fat cells become disproportionately larger, and en masse, are visible as unsightly bulges. The interesting thing about fat cells is that the number of fat cells does not increase during your lifespan. Essentially, you are born with the number of fat cells that you will die with, (unless, of course, you have some removed through liposuction). As you put on weight and increase in size, the fat cells that you have increase in size, *but they do not multiply in number.*

This is in clear contradistinction to skin cells, where your skin cells are rapidly multiplying all the time from the basal cell layer and migrating to the skin surface. When these cells reach the skin surface, 90 to 120 days later, they have already gone through their life cycle of birth and death during their travel from the basal or germinal layer, to the surface of the skin where in their dead state, they are called the keratin layer. This keratin layer, in people with very dry skin, can be visible as scaling patches that can be scratched off. In people with normal skin while this dead layer is not quite so clearly visible, it is nevertheless present, and represents the body's first line of defense against injury and intrusion.

The skin that you have today is not the skin you had four months ago. It is a brand new covering, admittedly with the same genetic origin, so that you look the same as you did four months ago, but nevertheless a brand new skin. In fact you are constantly shedding your old skin to be replaced by new skin. This shedding is obviously not as dramatic as in some animal species, such as snakes, where the skin is shed whole as one piece. However, you are shedding your skin all the time and simultaneously giving birth to new skin, which replaces the old.

Unlike skin, fat cells lack this genetic ability to multiply and simply increase in volume and size as they accumulate and store fat. Remember the purpose of these cells is simply to act as storage units for fat until that fat needs to be mobilized as an energy source in time of need when the cell should release the fat into the bloodstream to be utilized as an energy source. In patients seeking finesse liposuction the problem is that, in the areas which bother the patient, the fat cells have a high affinity for fat, which means that essentially when there is any fat available in the bloodstream those fat cells grab it first, in preference to the other fat cells in the body.

Conversely these fat cells are the last ones to let go of the fat even in times of need. This explains the common tale that these patients will tell when they come into the office, "Doctor a few years ago I didn't have these bulges and now, no matter what I do, they seem to be getting bigger and bigger. In fact when I exercise and diet I seem to lose weight from everywhere but these problem areas. And if, God forbid, I put any weight on it seems to go straight to those areas where I am desperately trying to lose it from!"

If this is your story then you are the ideal candidate for liposuction! I can tell you right now that no amount of exercise or dieting will get rid of those bulges if this is how you describe the problem that affects you. The only way to get rid of them is to remove the underlying fat through liposuction. The finesse in this kind of liposuction involves leaving just enough fat cells to achieve a normal contour and the ability to do that is where the artistry and expertise of the surgeon comes in. It takes a lot more artistry and skill to perform finesse liposuction than liposuction for volume where the essential goal is simply to remove as much volume of fat as possible consistent with the patient's safety.

To illustrate all that I have just said about liposuction let me tell you about Sarah. She came to see me because she was very conscious about the size of her ankles. Now for men reading, "Doctor, Is Liposuction Right for Me?" this may not seem like the most obvious area to start, but believe me, for women the size of their ankles is a big deal! However more importantly this case illustrates several important points about liposuction.

Firstly, it exposes the myth that you can achieve selective weight loss by exercising the affected area. It is impossible to overestimate how widespread this myth is. The reality is that no matter how many leg lifts or ankle exercises Sarah performs, and her overall condition and tone testified to her daily workouts, this will do nothing to the layer of fat directly overlying these muscles that she is working out. The same applies to fat deposits on the outer and inner thighs, and around the knees. Similarly, in the face, no matter what exercises you do with neck or jaw muscles, those exercises are not going to translate into the improved jaw and necklines that can be achieved with an hours worth of finesse liposuction!

Once I explained this concept of high affinity fat receptors that result in these deposits of unwanted and unsightly fat it became self-evident to Sarah that all the hours in the gym on the stair-master could never possibly correct the shape of her ankles and calves and she elected to have the surgery as soon as possible.

Her post-operative results at three months achieved an excellent change in her ankle and calves, but it really did require the full three months for the skin to shrink to the contours of her new shape. During this period the nerves that provide sensation to the skin of her calf and ankle were quite numb because these nerves are so superficial and have little protection from the liposuction cannula which, while it cannot suction out the nerves because of their different consistency from fat can, nevertheless, cause sufficient injury to these nerves to send them into a prolonged period of shock from which they did not recover for a full three months.

The analogy I have found most useful in explaining what happens to the nerves in the areas that are liposuctioned to patients is to compare it to what happens when you cross your legs and the leg falls "asleep". This is due to the very brief period of pressure on the affected nerve from the weight of the crossed leg. When you uncross the leg, the nerve begins to recover and you get a feeling of pins and needles in the leg, which is the manifestation of the nerve recovering and very rapidly these pins and needle feelings go away as the nerve recovers completely. Well, in liposuction, it is not very brief external pressure that is affecting the nerves but rather repeated attacks on these nerves, which run in the fat, from the liposuction cannula. The more exposed and superficial these nerves run, as in the calf and ankle, the more exposed they are to injury during liposuction and the longer they take to return to normal. But, as I pointed out earlier, thick ankles and calves are sufficiently bothersome to female patients that they will accept the prolonged recovery period involved in liposuction of the ankles and calves. In areas such as the abdomen and flanks and thighs where the nerves are more protected the sensation of pins and needles is not so bothersome because the nerves run deeper and are more protected.

The most common areas, where patients request finesse liposuction are the outer and inner thighs. This, also, is an area where females more commonly request liposuction than males because of the different patterns of fat distribution in the sexes. These ladies suffer from disproportion so that when they go shopping they have to buy separates with a larger size of pants and a smaller size of the coordinating blouse or top. If this describes you, and you are at, or near, your ideal body weight, you are almost certainly a good candidate for finesse liposuction.

Fat contouring of the inner knees is also something requested, almost exclusively, by females and removal of small deposits of fat can make significant changes in the shape of the knees. This is often done at the same time as the inner thighs are worked on, and can significantly slenderize the leg. Results here can be very rapidly visible, and provide an immediate and gratifying change.

Finesse liposuction is also extremely popular with bodybuilders and fitness buffs, who through exercise and work-out have excellent muscles for their efforts, but wish added definition of these muscles by removing a small subcutaneous layer of fat, so that the muscles show through the skin even more. This is an excellent role for finesse liposuction and the results are rapidly visible to both patient and surgeon, not to mention the other members of the gym!

The most dramatic use of liposuction for finesse is in the face and neck. In about one hour the surgeon can contour a more youthful face and neckline through minimal incisions and can result in amazing changes in patients both young and old. One of the reasons why finesse liposuction of the face and neck is extremely successful is that unlike other areas of the body, where we have to wait for the skin to shrink to see the final result, in the neck we actually need more skin to cover the deeper neck line. The result is visible to the patient almost as soon as the swelling from the surgery has subsided. I'm always happy to see a patient that wants liposuction of the neck in the office because it really is one of the most gratifying operations to perform and gives superb results.

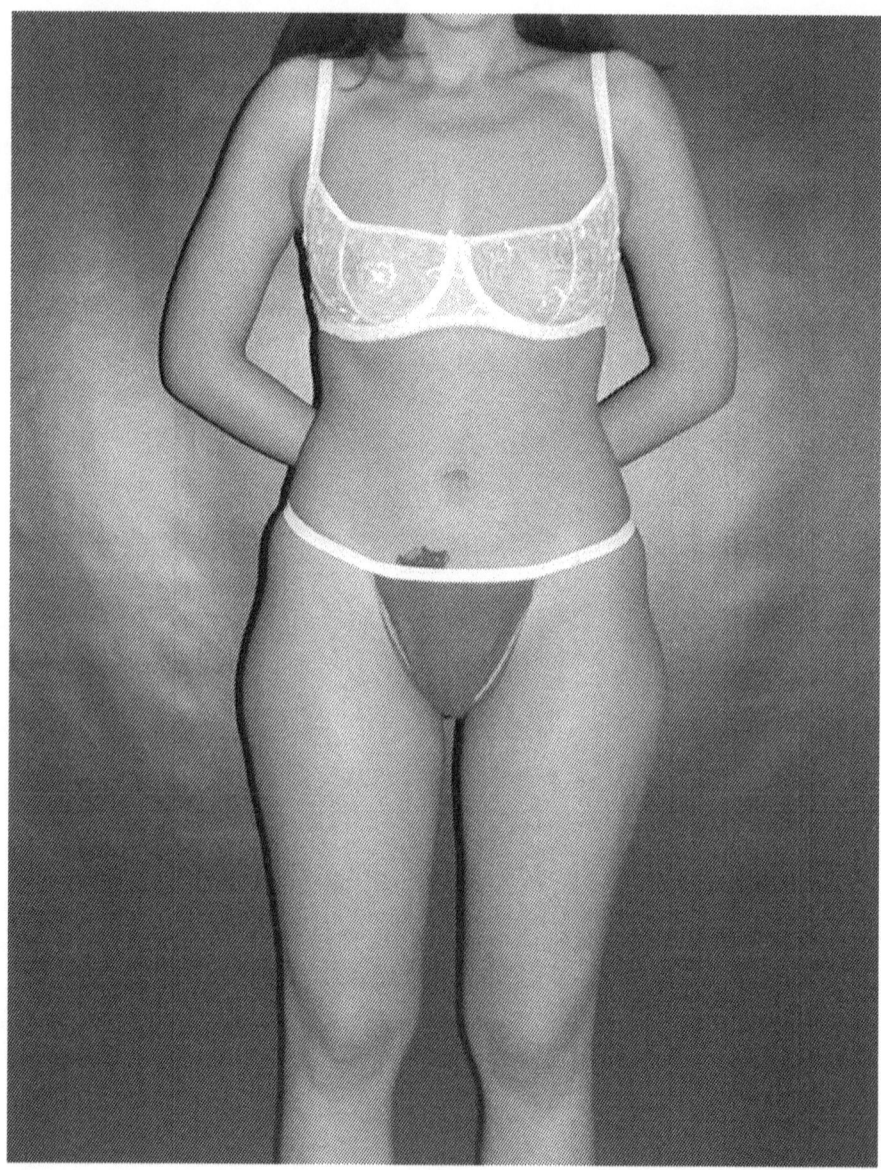

**Figure 6.1: Andrea pre-operatively before finesse liposuction of the outer thighs.**

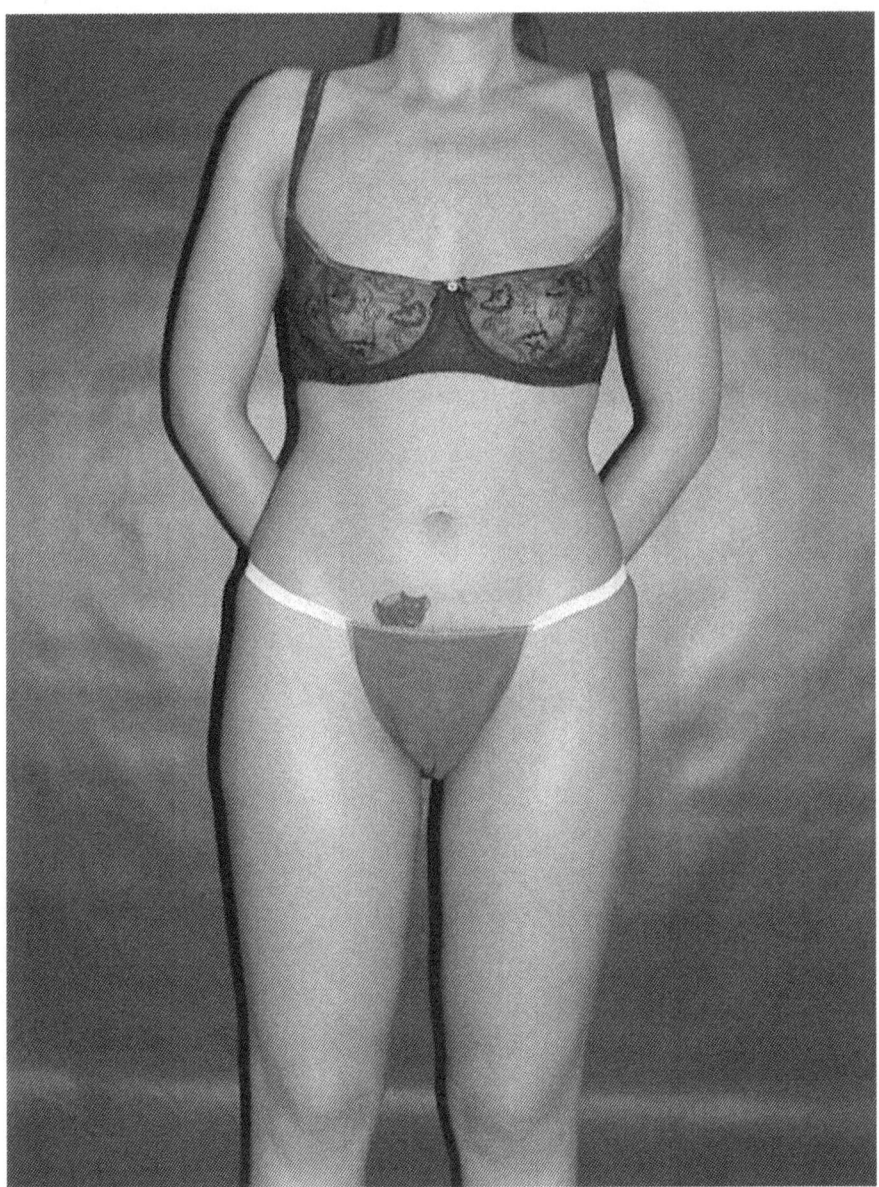

Figure 6.2: Andrea post-operatively after finesse liposuction of the outer thighs. Note how the entire body now is in proportion.

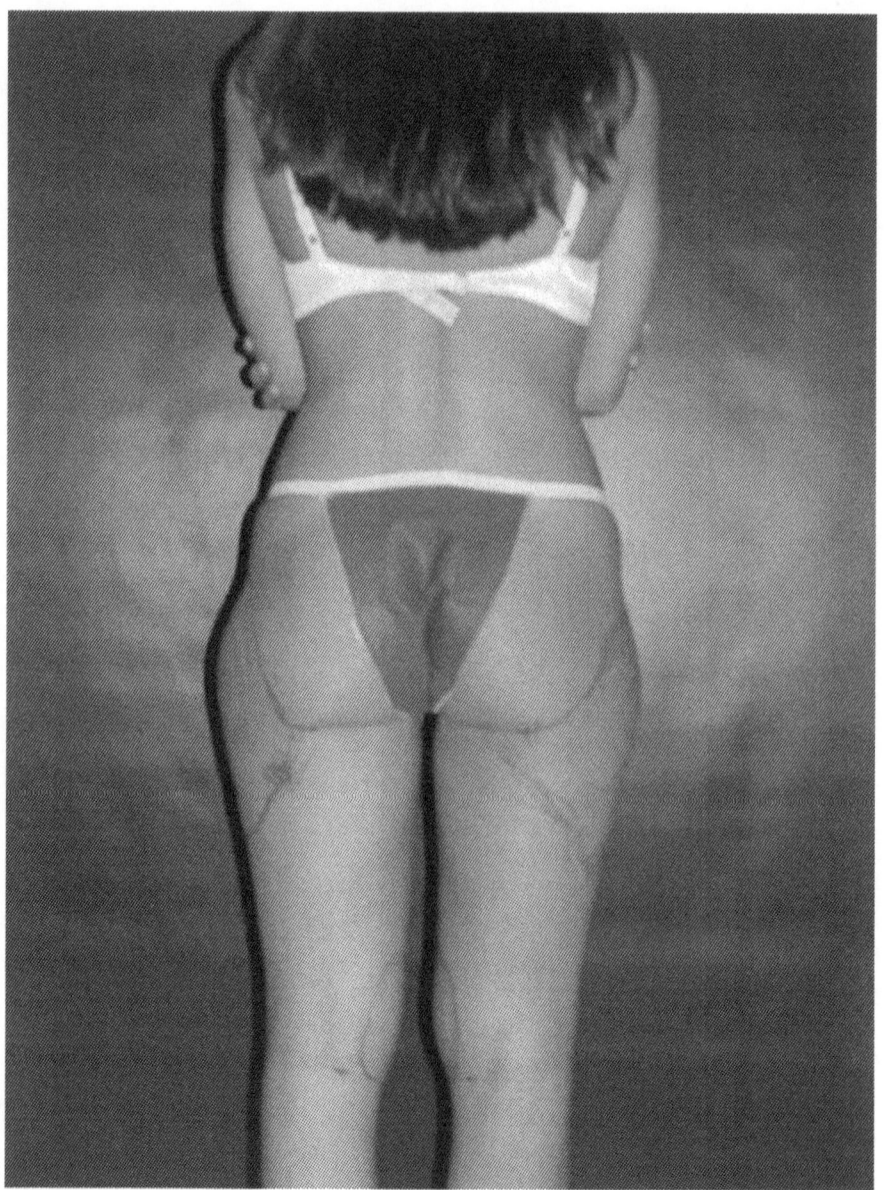

Figure 6.3: Andrea pre-operatively showing the markings for finesse liposuction of the outer thighs and inner knees.

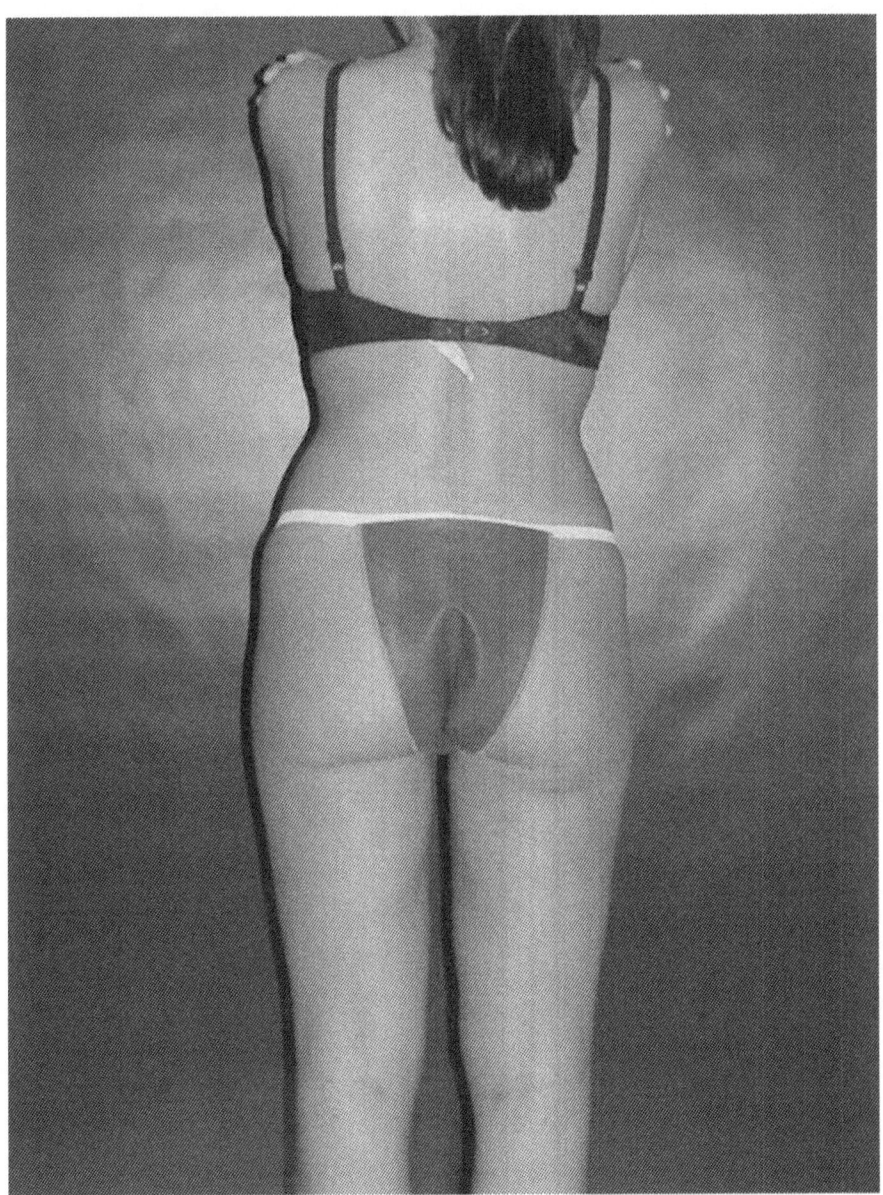

Figure 6.4: Andrea post-operatively after finesse liposuction of the inner kneepads and outer thighs.

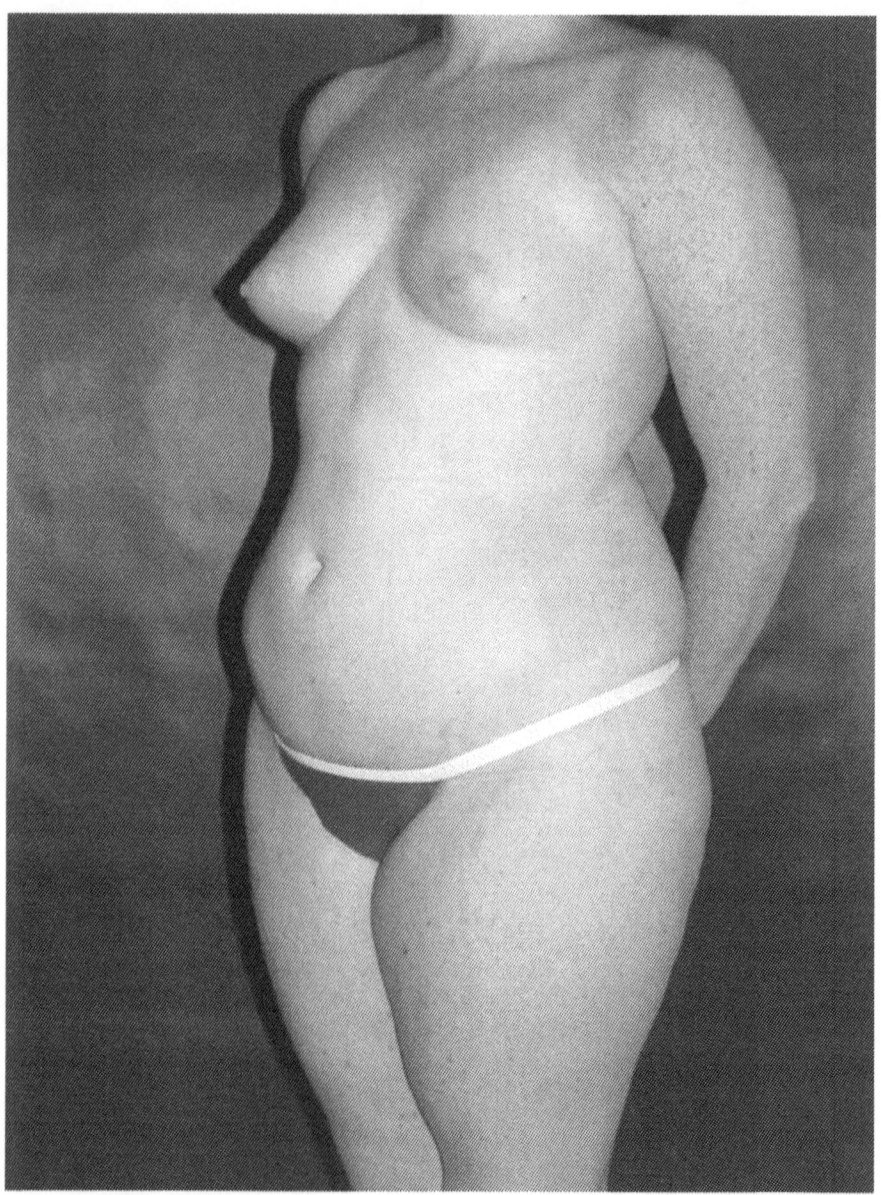

Figure 6.5: Bernadette prior to finesse liposuction of the abdomen. At the same procedure she had volume liposuction of the back (see Figure 7.1)

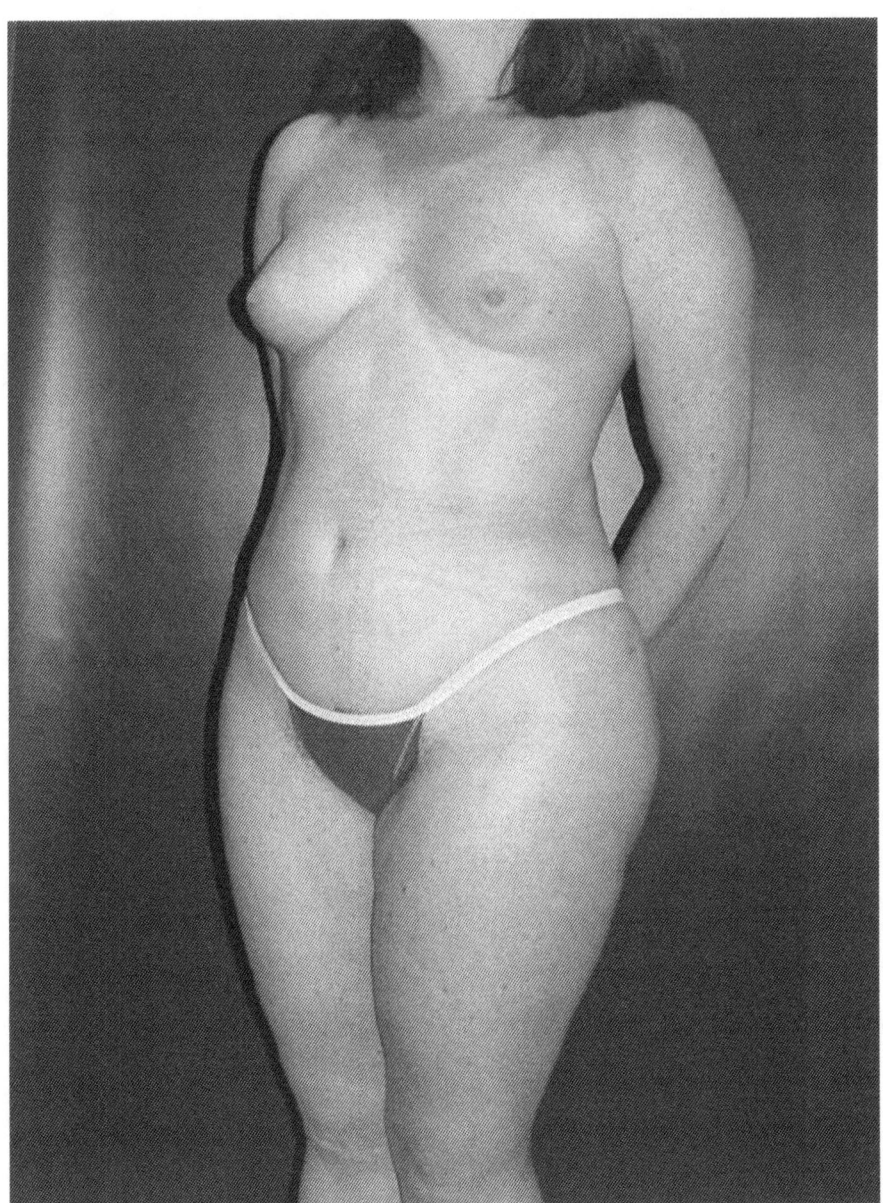

Figure 6.6: Bernadette after finesse liposuction of the abdomen.

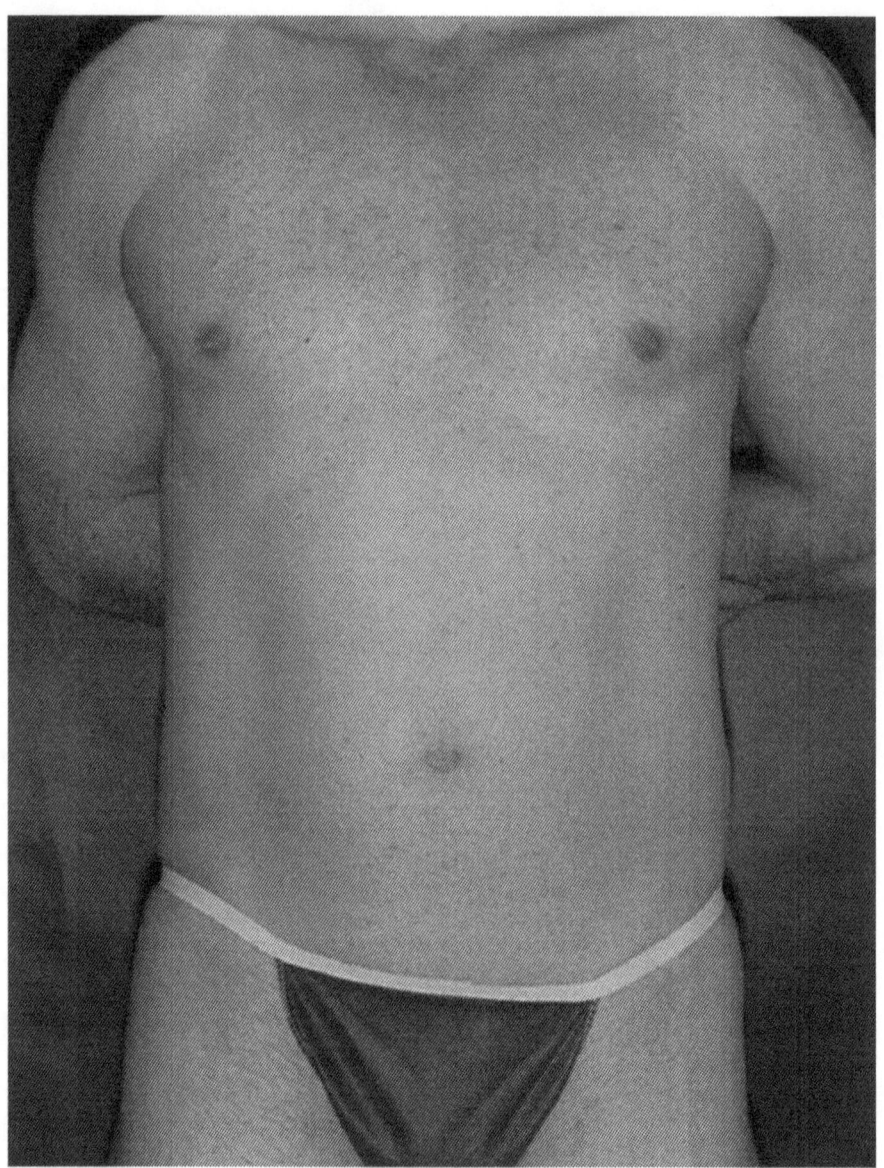

Figure 6.7: Charles, a personal trainer, works out in the gym at least two hours a day but is still not able to achieve the muscle definition he is seeking.

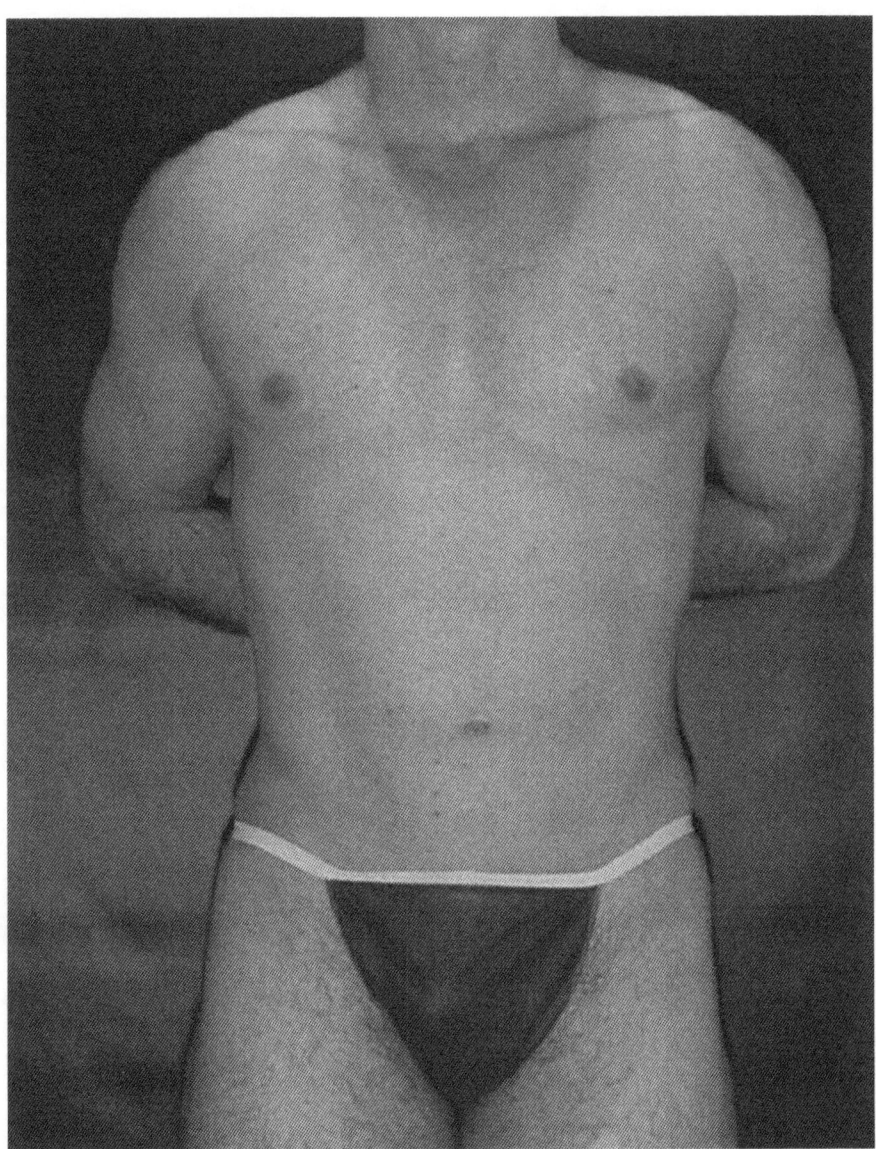

Figure 6.8: Charles, shortly after finesse liposuction of the abdomen. Note the tapering of the waistline and the better definition of the abdominal muscles. A clear testament to the fact that some changes cannot be achieved by working out alone!

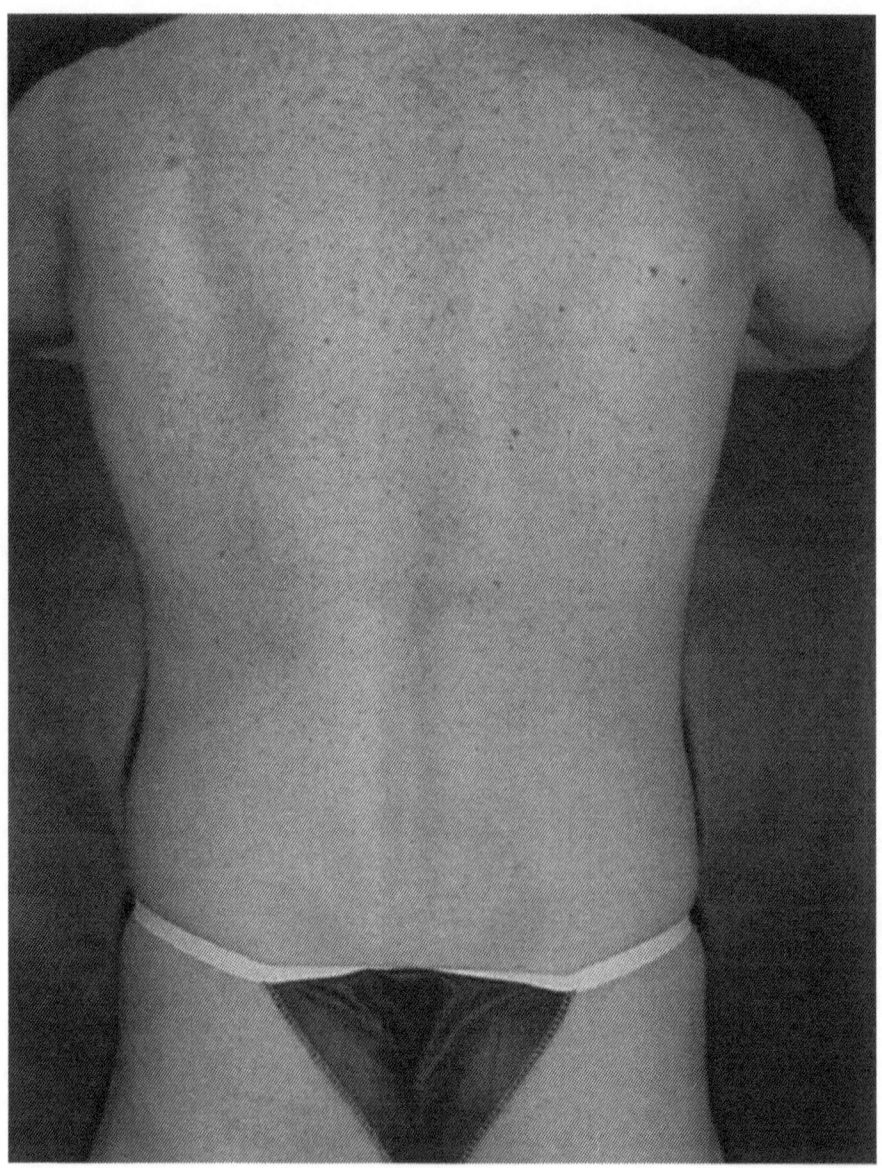

Figure 6.9: Charles, now seen from the back, pre-operatively, was also concerned about the lack of definition of his waistline.

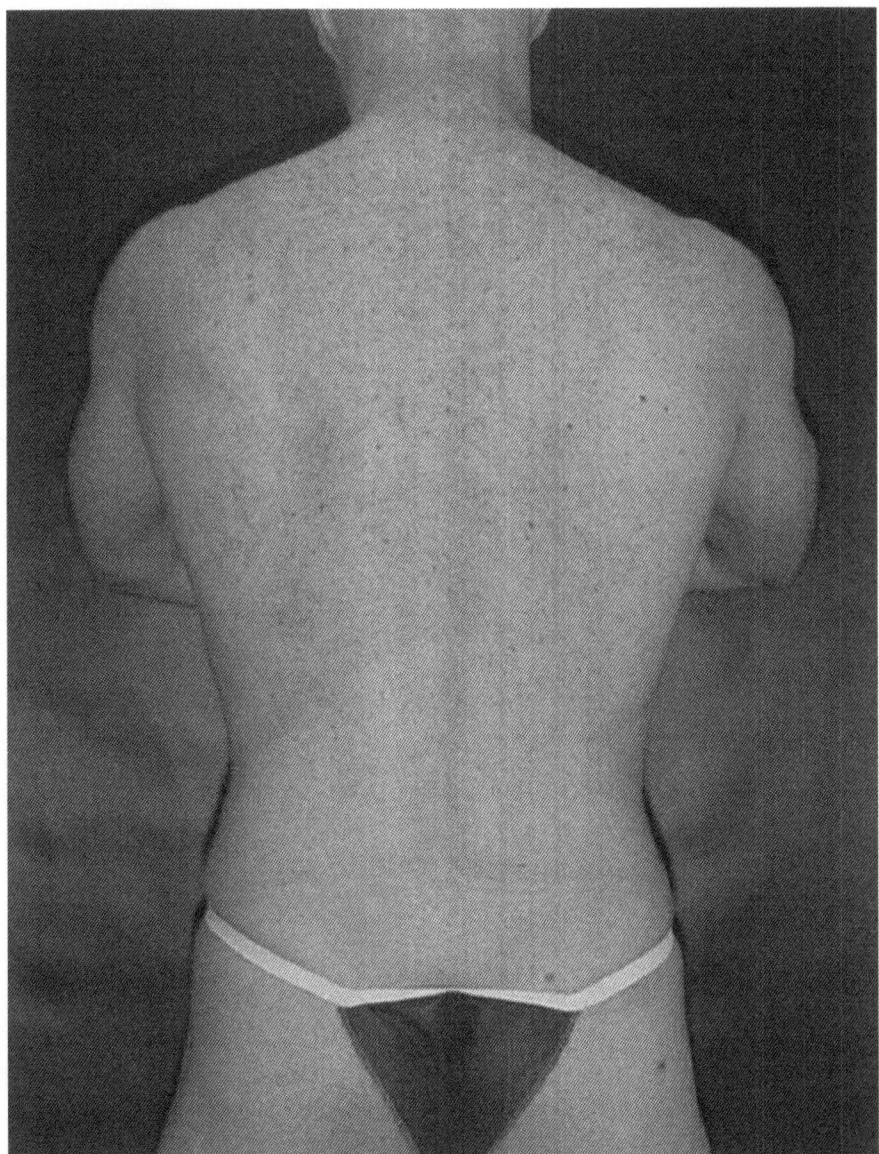

Figure 6.10: Charles, after finesse liposuction of his waistline, seen from behind. A dramatic reduction in the size of the waistline was achieved with only two hours of surgery.

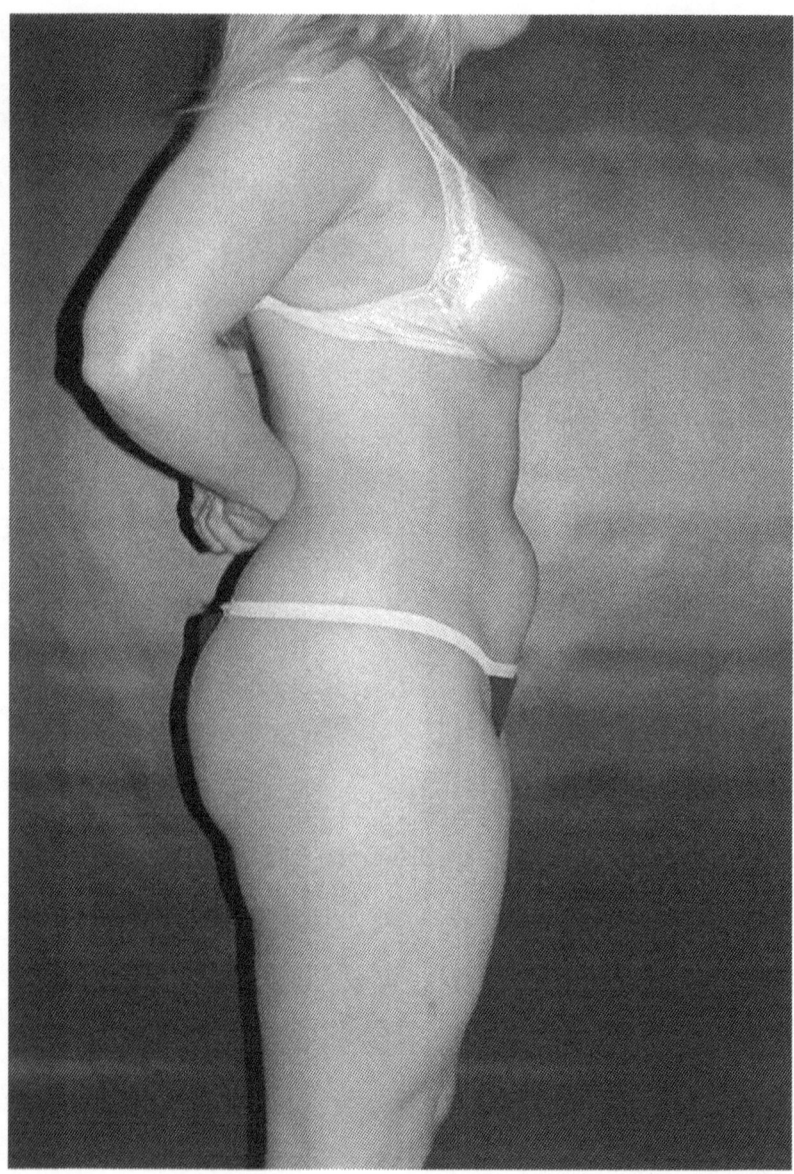

Figure 6.11: Deidra presented with a small amount of fat just below the umbilicus. This is a very common presentation of patients seeking finesse liposuction.

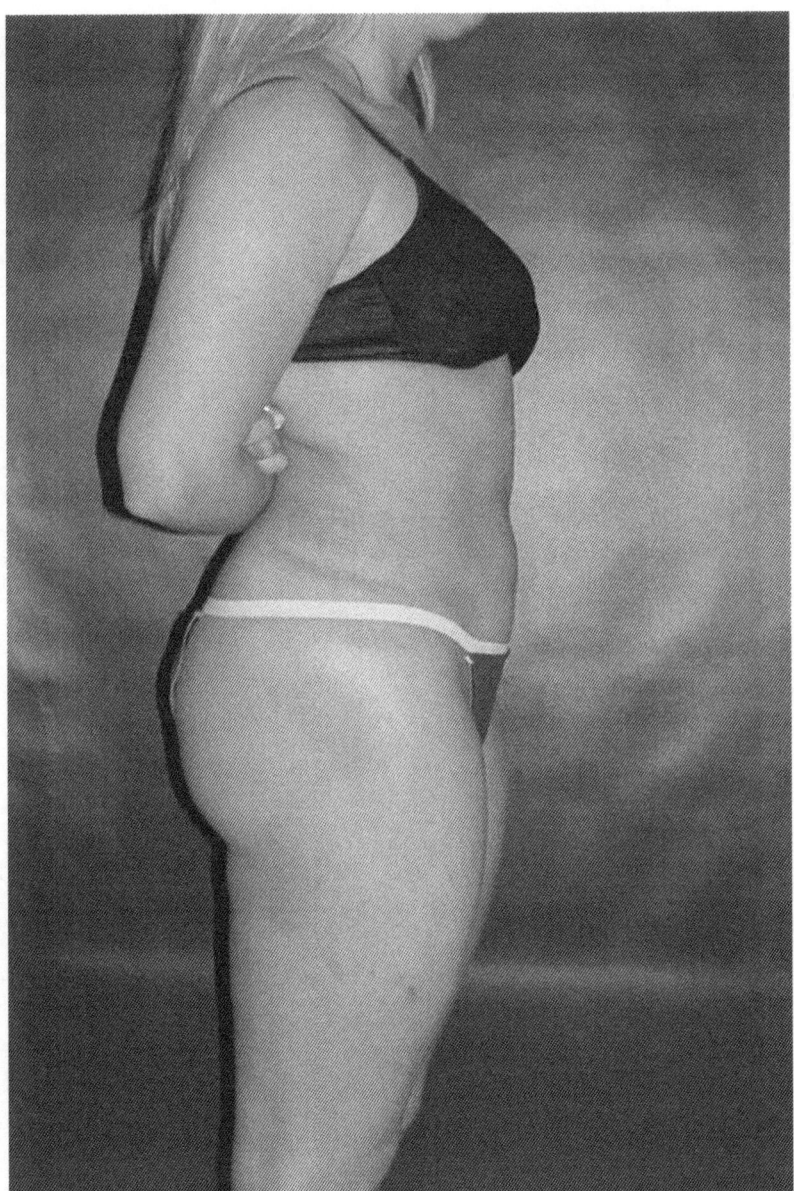

Figure 6.12: Deidra, after finesse liposuction of the lower abdomen, has a waistline proportional to the rest of her figure.

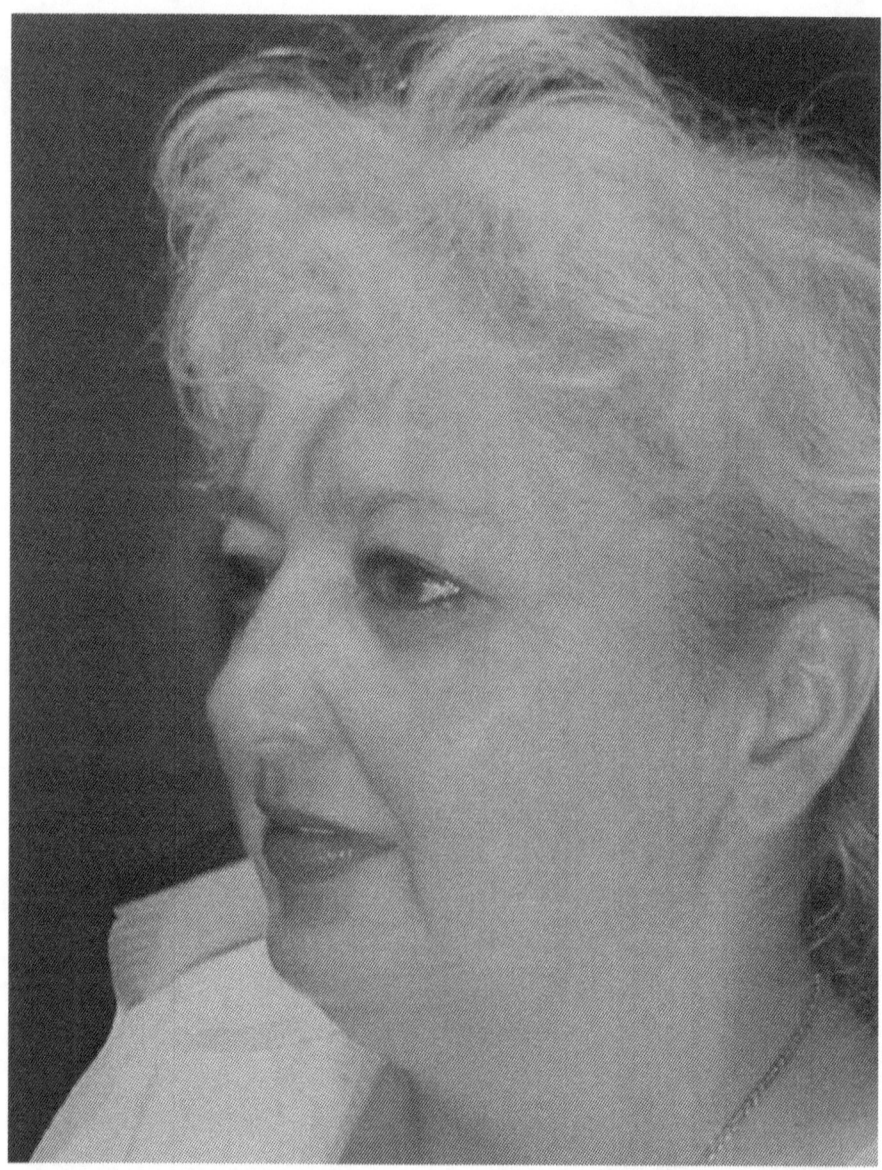

**Figure 6.13: Elizabeth sought consultation for her neckline and originally thought that a face-lift was the only solution to her problem.**

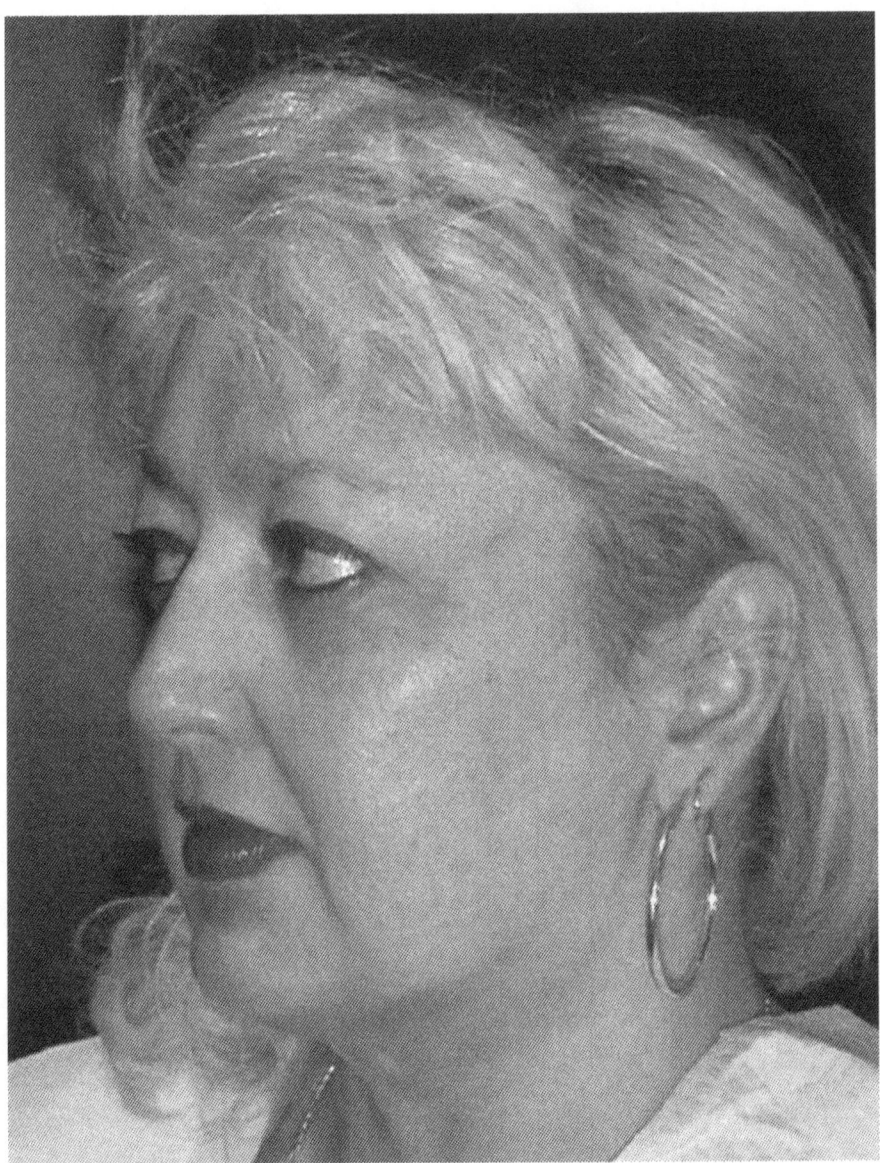

Figure 6.14: Elizabeth, after finesse liposuction of the neck and jaw line, was able to achieve the improvement she was looking for without a face-lift.

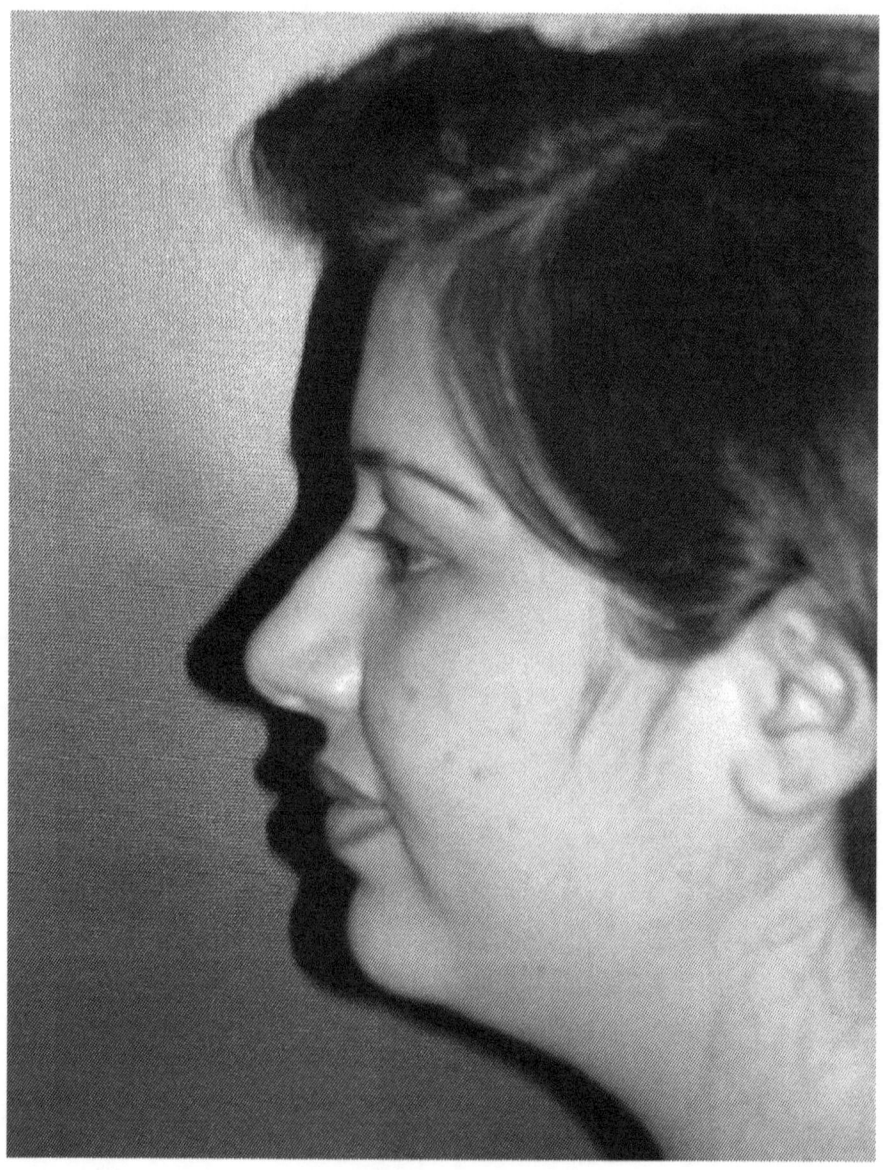

**Figure 6.15: Farrah, a much younger patient than Elizabeth, has the same neckline problem.**

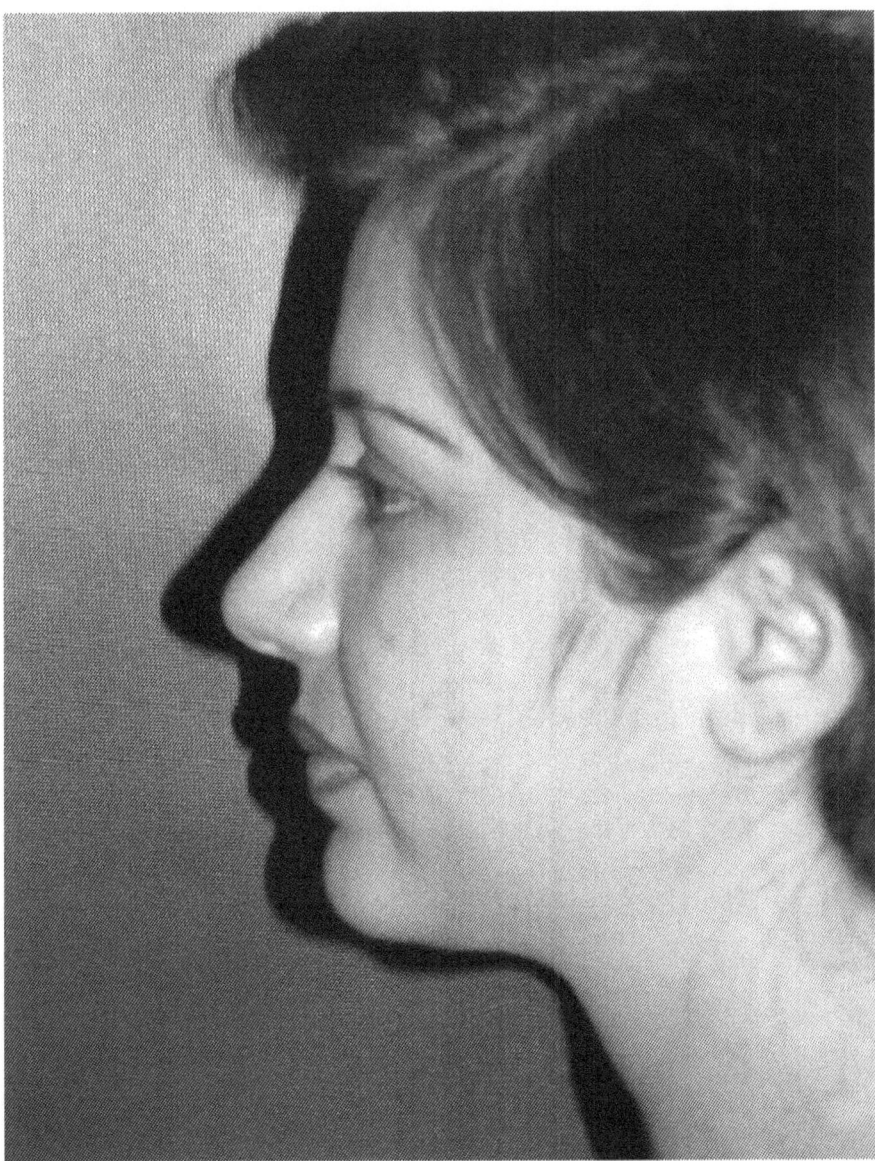

Figure 6.16: Farrah, post-operatively, with a much younger looking face achieved through finesse liposuction.

# Chapter 7

## Volume Liposuction

The patient who is overweight and consults with me about liposuction, usually regarding the abdomen, poses much more of a problem. In the previous chapter on finesse liposuction advising the patient was simple. For these patients there is simply no way to correct their problem other than liposuction. Almost always these patients are at or near their ideal bodyweight. In fact, I have performed finesse liposuction on some patients who were even below their ideal body weight and others who were marathon runners!

In the overweight patient, seeking liposuction for volume reduction, we have to confront a whole host of different questions. I have to confess here and now, that as someone who is prone to being overweight myself, that I have confronted these questions myself on a personal level. Having thought about this subject long and hard, I have come to the conclusion that there are no right or wrong answers. However, the following is the best advice that I can give and this usually helps the patients answer, for themselves, the question that is the title of this book: " Doctor, Is Liposuction Right for Me?"

If liposuction is attractive to the overweight patient as a potential "quick fix" to their problems then they need to be disabused of this notion. Liposuction has almost nothing to do with weight and is all about shape and form. While it is true that the additional fat the patient is carrying around gives rise to the shape and form that the patient wishes to change, and this avoirdupois has some heft it is far less than patients imagine. Looking back at the patients who had finesse liposuction, even when they had as much as 1.5 liters removed, (which should equate mathematically to a weight reduction of 3.3 lbs), these patients while they look better, their weight, on average, was unchanged. In my view this is explained by the fact that, since the body is seventy percent water, the fat removed from those unsightly areas has been replaced by water which, of course, is distributed evenly throughout the body and is not concentrated in any one specific area, such as the ankles or thighs from where the fat was removed.

Furthermore, in the patients who sought finesse liposuction, their problem was related to the concept of high affinity fat receptors causing their problem of disproportion. This concept cannot be applied to those patients who are simply overweight. There are no specific set of fat cells with high affinity fat receptors giving rise to their problem! The inevitable truth is that these patients are consuming more calories than they are spending on a daily basis and their body is simply responding by storing the excess calories, for time of need, in the form of fat.

I explained the problem exactly this way to a significantly overweight preacher who had come to see me regarding liposuction and after digesting this information he said to me, "You know, Doctor, in the Bible it is talked about the seven years of plenty being followed by the seven years of lean. It's just that in modern day America that famine never seems to come!" To this day that is probably the best description I have heard of what losing weight entails: a self-imposed famine.

Now, let me be clear, I am not unsympathetic to the patient's problems. In fact, as I said earlier on, as someone who is prone to putting on weight myself, I have had to face these problems myself. And if a preacher, a man of the cloth, is disturbed by being overweight, just imagine how much more difficult it is for a plastic surgeon like myself!

The problem then, is that while volume liposuction will make a significant reduction in the patient's size, it is not a solution to the problem of excess calorie intake, which caused the problem in the first place! Unlike the patient undergoing finesse liposuction, where we can anticipate a permanent solution to their problem, the patient considering volume liposuction can expect that the surgery will aid them towards their goal but, by itself, liposuction will not solve their problem. If these patients can accept liposuction as an important adjunct to their diet and exercise program then they are candidates for liposuction. If they expect the liposuction to do it all, then they will be sorely disappointed in the results of the surgery. These are the patients who have given liposuction a bad rap. Patients who have come into my office would often say something like, "I had a friend who had liposuction and it just didn't work for her. She put the weight right back on!"

My point precisely! You _can_ put it back on and it is all too easy to do just that, if you don't maintain a rigorous diet and exercise program. Fortunately, most of the patients I see considering liposuction for volume are well aware that the surgery will not "cure" their problem, and that while the surgery is not a substitute for diet and exercise, it can be a significant help to them in achieving their goals.

This is best illustrated by looking at some pictures. On first inspection, patient Jaclyn (Figs 7.15-20) did not look as if she was a candidate for liposuction. She looked as if she needed to lose weight. Initially, I was a little bit skeptical of her claims that she worked out daily for about two hours and was really controlling her diet. But on examination under the layers of fat I found her abdominal muscles were as firm as rock, and in fact, when you examine the pictures carefully, you can actually see the muscle outlines. It became increasingly clear to me as I listened to her that she was telling the truth, and that even with a rigorous diet and exercise program, this is where she had plateaued.

The results three months following surgery were phenomenal and everything I could have hoped for. The rock hard abdominal muscles that I had felt through the layers of fat were now clearly visible after the curtain of fat overlying them had been liposuctioned away. Clearly the patient had maintained a rigorous diet and exercise program and the smile on her face said it all in terms of how delighted she was with the result. The side views of Jaclyn show the impressive reduction in abdominal girth achieved. It was impossible to sufficiently tailor her old wardrobe of clothes to her new size but she was more than happy to get rid of them and go shopping for a whole new wardrobe of clothes!

A few months later Jaclyn was back in my office still in excellent shape and obviously very happy. I asked her how I could help her. "You might think this is strange Doctor", she said, "But I still have fat that I can pinch and I was wondering if you could go back in and take more out?" On a purely mechanical level the answer is simple. If you can pinch the fat between your thumb and index finger, then you can remove that fat with liposuction.

The more important question is: Will I make the patient happy by doing so? And that is really a question only the patient can answer for him or herself. Many patients would be more than happy with the shape that Jaclyn achieved from her first surgery just as many people will look at patients undergoing finesse liposuction and say, "Really these people don't need liposuction. I would be more than happy if I looked like that."

This brings us to another truism in cosmetic surgery. The more attractive the patient is, the more cognizant they are of any minor imperfections. Sometimes, when an extremely attractive patient comes in and wants the tip of their nostril lifted just a millimeter or collagen injections to define the border of their lips, it is possible to point out to patients that the rest of the world is just not going to notice the difference, and in fact, only by carefully scrutinizing the pre and post procedure pictures can the subtle changes achieved be noted.

Essentially what Jaclyn was seeking, now that she had successfully benefited from volume liposuction was to have even more improvement, this time from finesse liposuction. The answer to her question, of course, is yes, because quite simply, if she had presented initially with the great shape she now had, she would have been a candidate for finesse liposuction. Why should the fact that she had utilized volume liposuction to get to this point be held against her? As long as the areas she wanted liposuctioned had recovered from the initial surgery, you can always go back and take more out if you can pinch the fat between your thumb and index finger. In fact, this kind of staged liposuction is something that is extremely successful because it allows the skin to contract sequentially and if you turn now and look at the result achieved by the second procedure for Jaclyn (Figs 7.15-20) it is clear that result could never have been achieved in one operation. Firstly, she could not have withstood the trauma of losing that much of her body in one operation. Secondly, I doubt if the skin could possibly have contracted as much in one stage as it was able to do in two stages.

The shrinkage of the skin is critical to the final result because even if the bulges of fat are gone if the visible result is skin that did not shrink smoothly and evenly then the end result will not be attractive. Patients understand this intuitively and the larger the volume of liposuction the more the skin has to contract so staging volume liposuction procedures is highly recommended for this reason as well as the fact that it is simply safer.

Jaclyn is not the typical patient to illustrate the goals of volume liposuction. The goals of most patients are much more limited and a more typical patient is Ian (Figs. 7.11-14). At forty-four, he was a successful mid-level executive, but felt that his size was standing in the way of further advancement up the corporate ladder. He was a big guy and his chest size as measured by the suit that he was wearing was 46inches and his pant size was 49 inches. Standing five foot ten inches tall he weighed in at over 210 lbs. The insurance tables said he should be no more than 170lbs.

When he came into the office he was unsure wether he was really a candidate for liposuction and had come in more out of desperation than expectation. He related his story that despite exercising and controlling his diet he had not been able to make any headway in changing the shape of his body or losing any weight at all. The first thing that I explained to him was that even if I removed four liters of fat, almost certainly, his weight would not change because his body, sensing that loss, would hold onto four liters of water which weighs exactly the same as fat!

If he were to have surgery the goal would not be weight reduction but to make his abdomen more proportionate for his chest size. The other thing I was able to explain to him was that the standard weight tables just did not apply to him! The standard weight tables do not take into account the fact that two people of the same height may have very different chest sizes, which will result in very different body proportions and weight. Ian, with a 46inch chest, will obviously weigh in significantly heavier than someone of the same height who has a 38inch chest. This chest size is related not to fat but the size of the bony frame of the shoulders and the rib cage so clearly the person with a 38 inch chest will weigh less than Ian with a 46 inch chest, *even if they both have the same percentage body fat.*

More important to Ian's body proportion, given the fact that his chest size is essentially a fixed number, is what my tailor, Richard Cintron, refers to as *"the drop"*. In tailoring terminology the drop refers to the difference between the chest size and the waist size. In the standard American suit this drop is six inches, so that a size 40inch jacket comes paired with a 34inch waist pant. In the more suave Italian cuts the same size 40inch jacket would come matched with a 33inch pant. In Ian's case with his 48inch chest, his waistline should have been 42inches to be proportionate. But as you can see from the photographs his waist was significantly bigger than his chest.

As Richard says in his inimitable way, "Doctor, they can come to you to tailor their body to fit their clothes or they can come to me and I'll tailor their clothes to fit the body!" As an aside, Richard will also tell you, that the easiest way to look fat is to wear clothes that are too small. Men in particular are reluctant to give up and move to larger pant sizes with the unsightly effect that their belly hangs over their waistline, making them look even bigger than they are. Looking at Ian's pictures even though he claimed his waist line was forty-five it's clear that his abdominal girth is greater than his chest circumference so he probably is trying to fit himself into pants that are too small for his size.

After discussing the pros and cons of surgery Ian was enthused to go ahead even though the goals we outlined for the surgery were much more moderate than he had initially hoped for when he came in for consultation. Nevertheless removing four liters of fat from the abdomen is a significant size reduction in abdominal girth. To put this in context just think of the reverse: what size would your pants have to be if they had to accommodate four one-liter soft drink bottles? If you look now at the result achieved for Ian in the three month follow-up pictures, you can see the impressive reduction in abdominal girth achieved. Just as important Ian used the impetus of the surgery to redouble his efforts with his exercise program and diet to drop almost 20lbs in weight. While he still has a 46 inch chest his waist is now 38 inches and he has to have his tailor take his pants in rather than let them out when he buys a new suit!

It's the proportions of the body that matter more than the absolute size. Patients who are heavy can be attractive as long as they are proportionate all over for their size. As evidence of this, just look at the female plus size models. They are attractive, even though by traditional standards they are overweight, because they are proportionate.

In conclusion, liposuction for volume can be very successful when combined with a diet and exercise program, but liposuction alone will have almost no effect on the weight of the patient, even though it will change the patient's shape. Like most other surgeons, though, I also have patients who had liposuction only to put the fat back on almost immediately. It is difficult pre-operatively to tell which patients really will stick to their promised exercise and diet program, and who will not, but the choice is theirs. After investing so much money, time and effort in liposuction, many patients are really motivated to maintain and enhance their new body through diet and exercise. *The patients who do so are some of the happiest in my practice.*

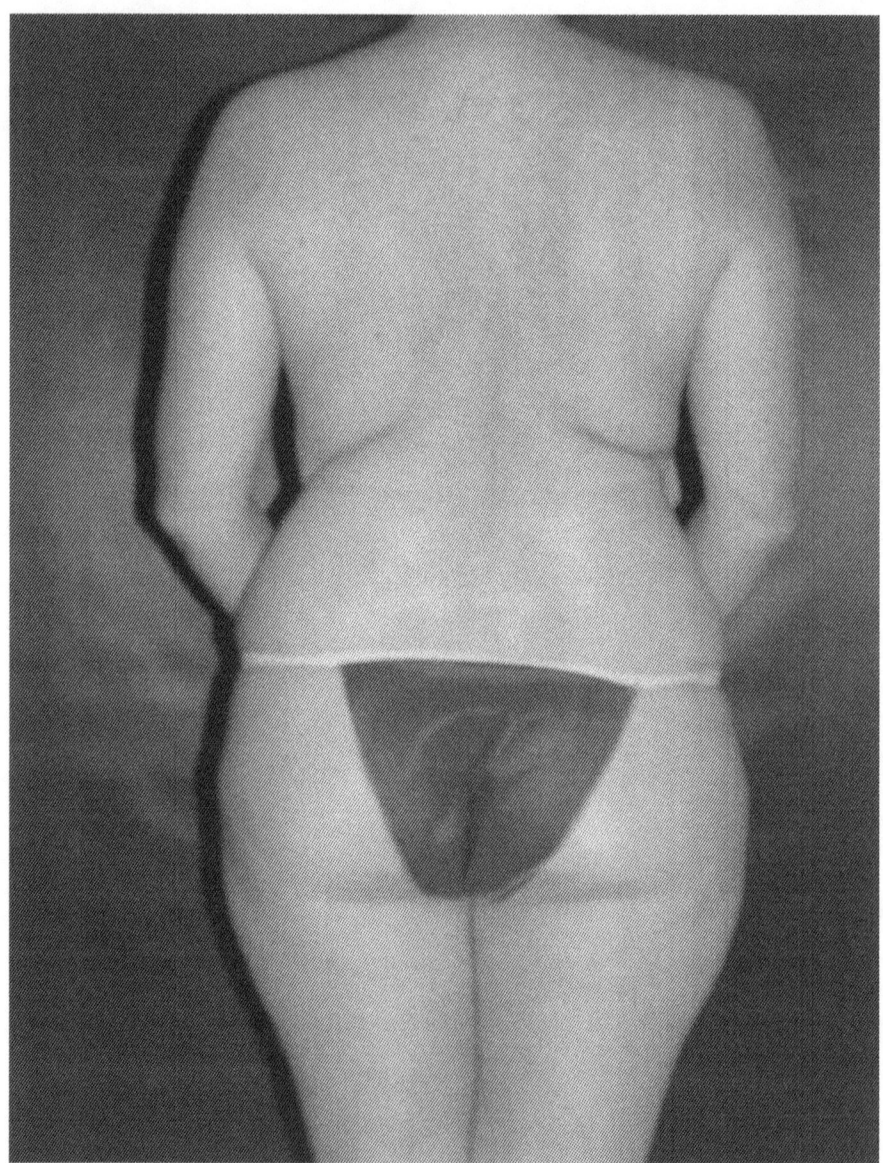

Figure 7.1: Bernadette, (the same patient as in Fig 6.5), from behind. While she only needed finesse liposuction of the abdomen, her back required volume reduction.

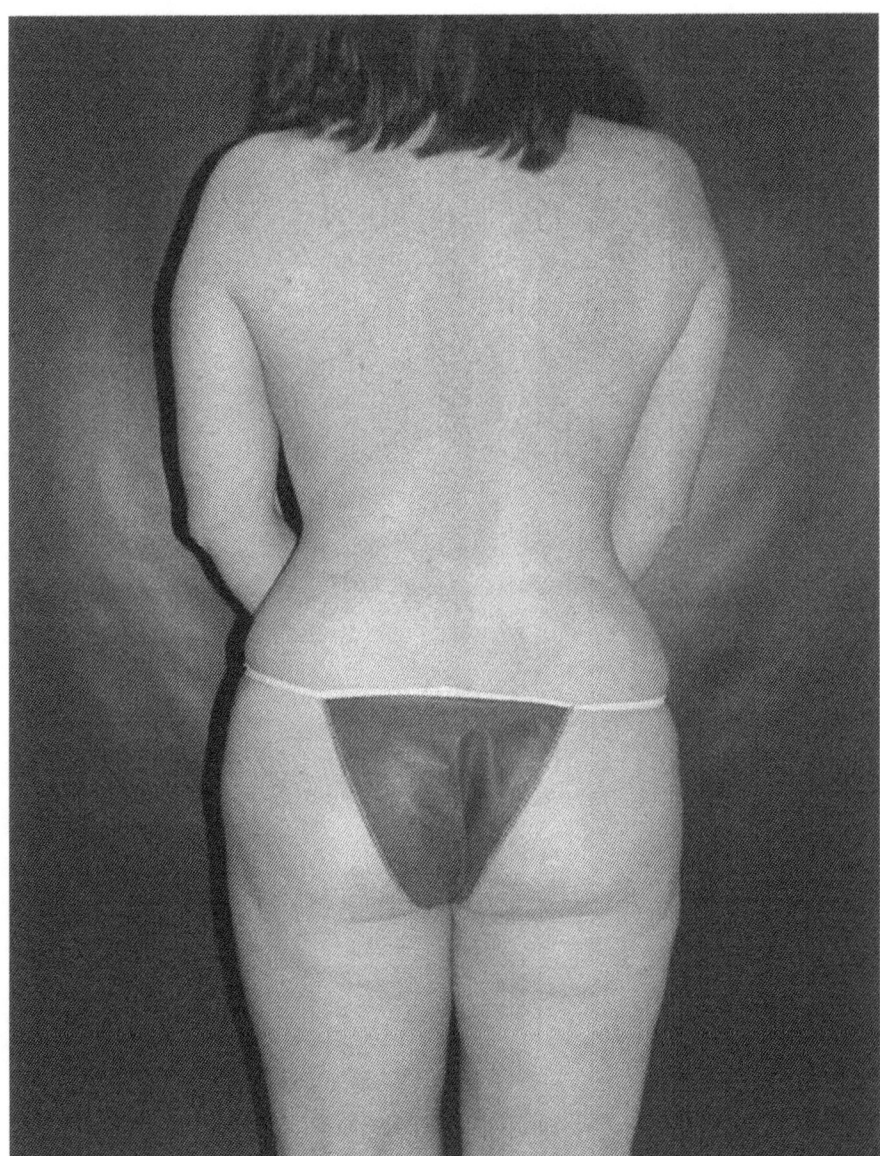

Figure 7.2: Bernadette's post-operative view shows a dramatic change in the post-operative size of the waist following liposuction for volume reduction.

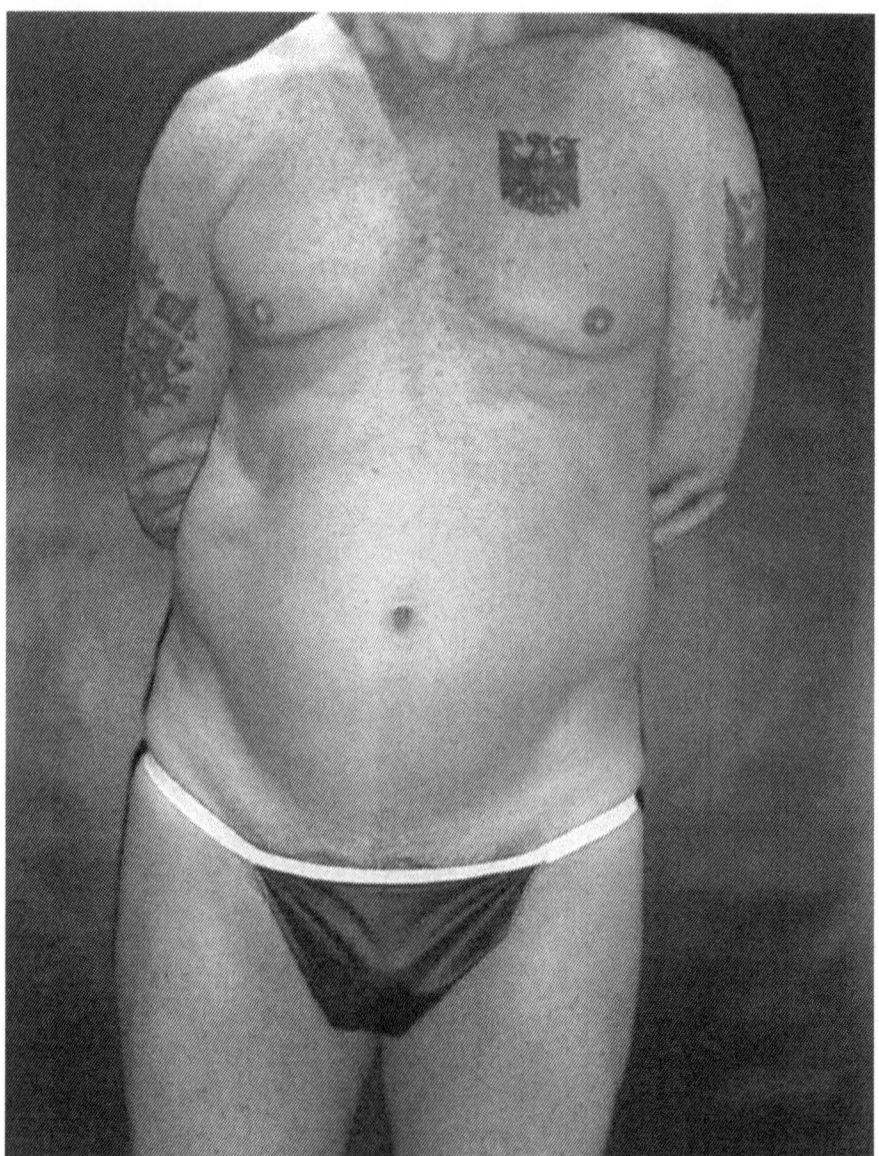

**Figure 7.3:** George, retired from the military, has been unable to get rid of his stomach paunch despite exercising daily.

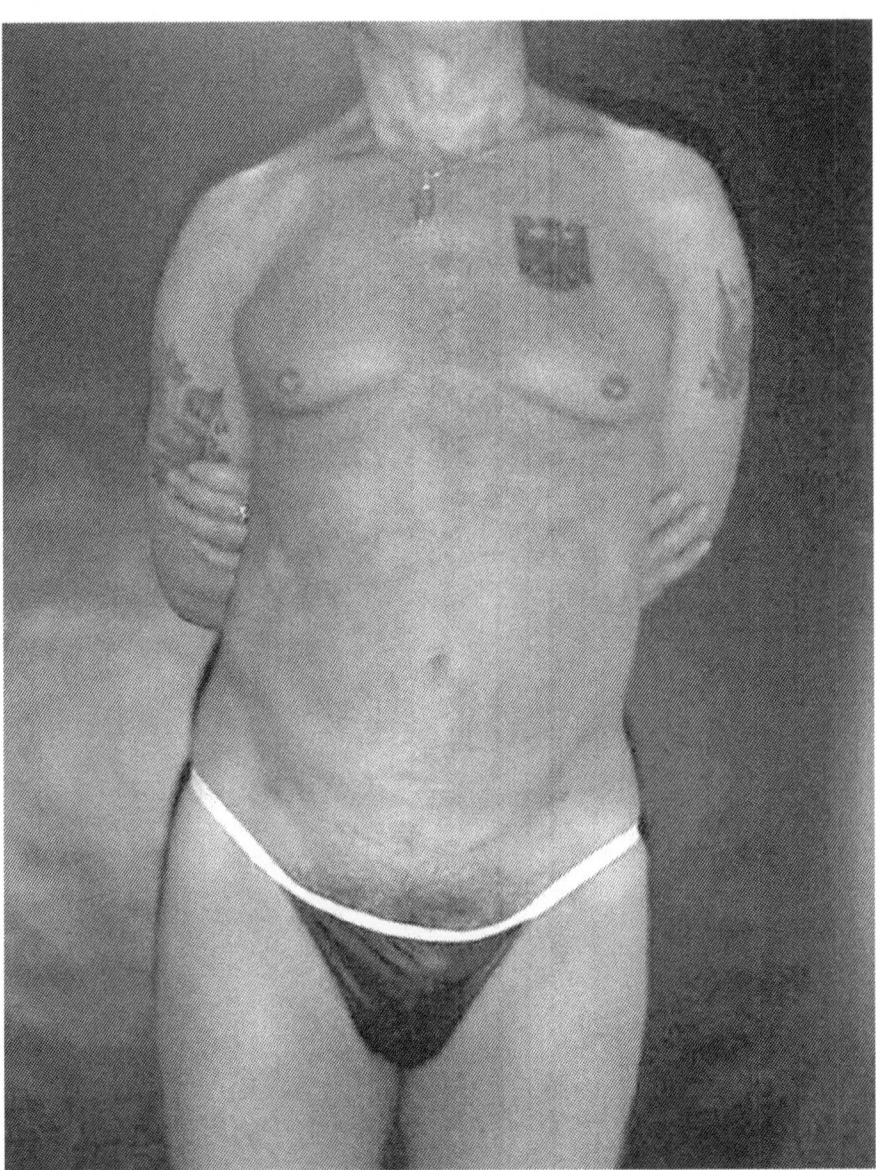

Figure 7.4: After a significant volume liposuction notice how well George's skin has shrunk to show his new, slimmer midriff.

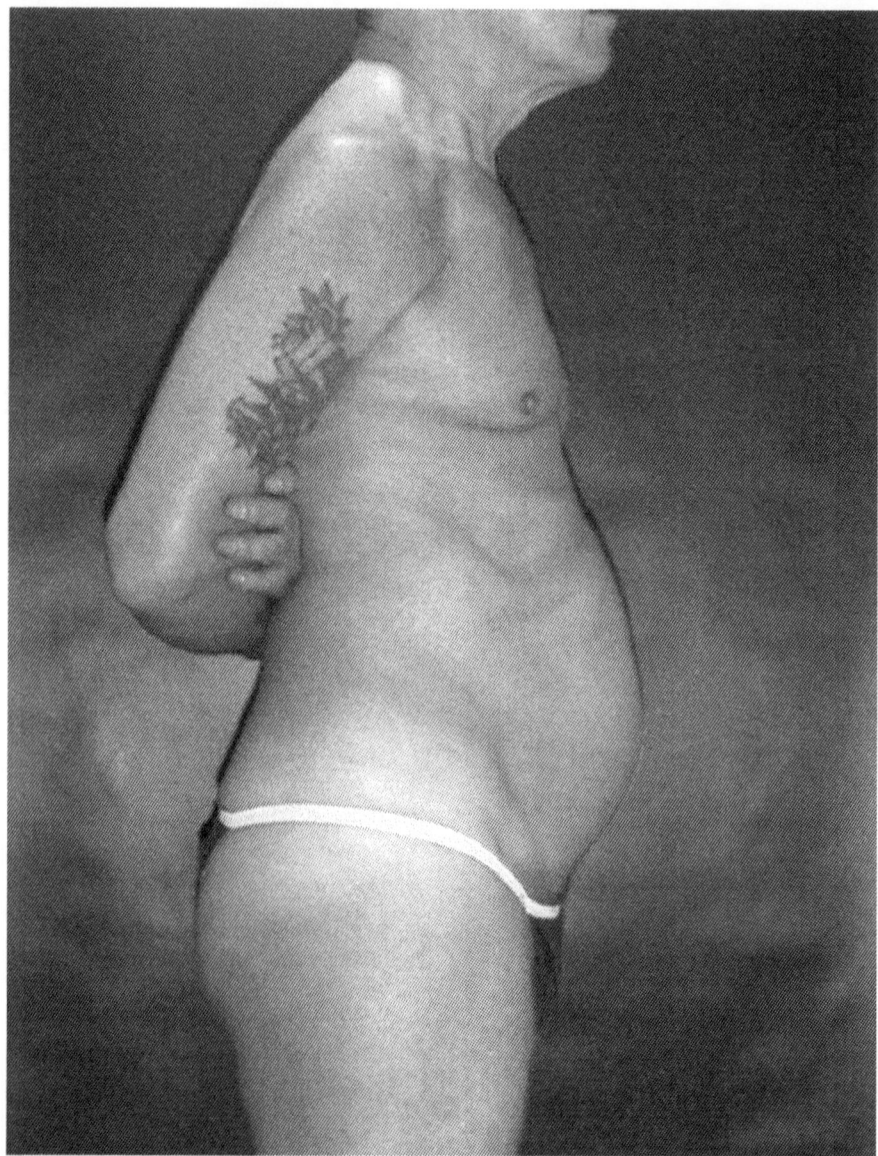

**Figure 7.5: George, pre-operatively, from the side view showing that his abdomen girth is significantly greater than his chest girth.**

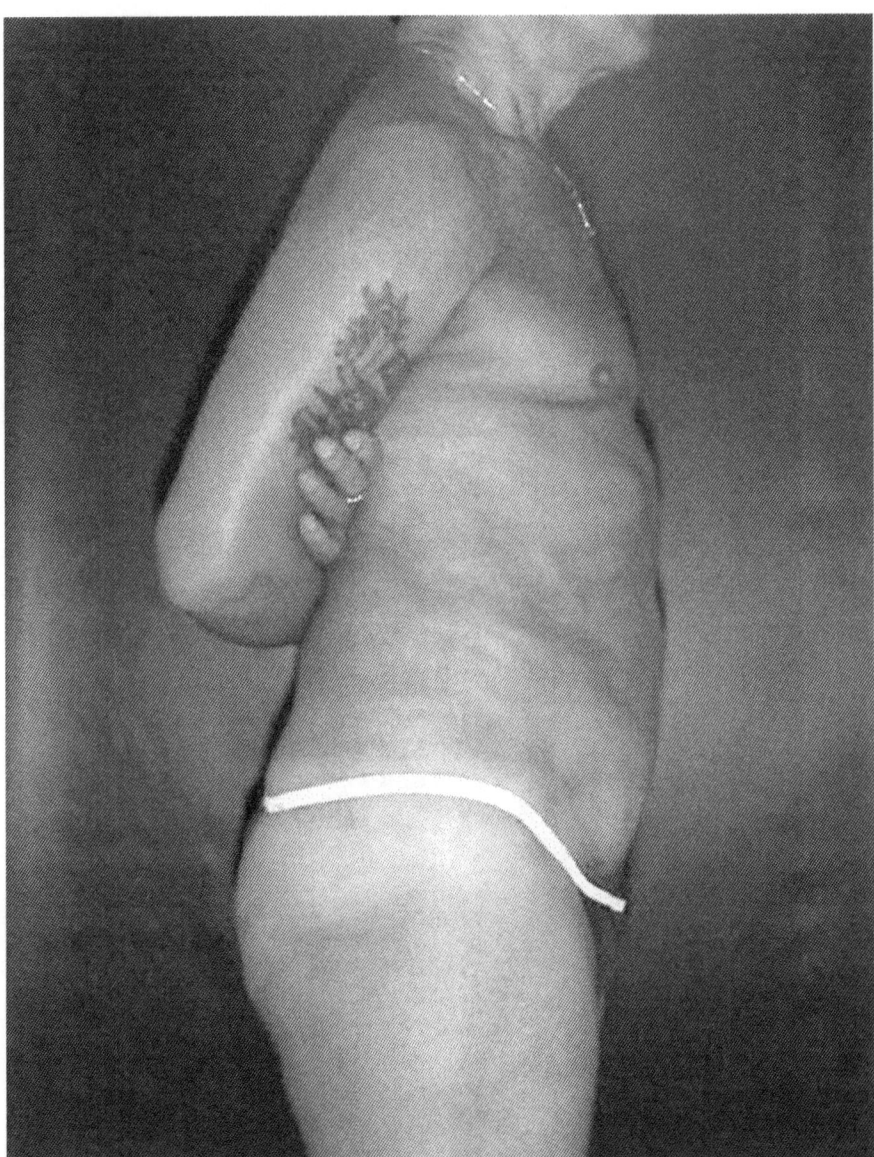

Figure 7.6: Post-operative picture shows the stomach paunch gone and George's waistline is now proportionate to his chest.

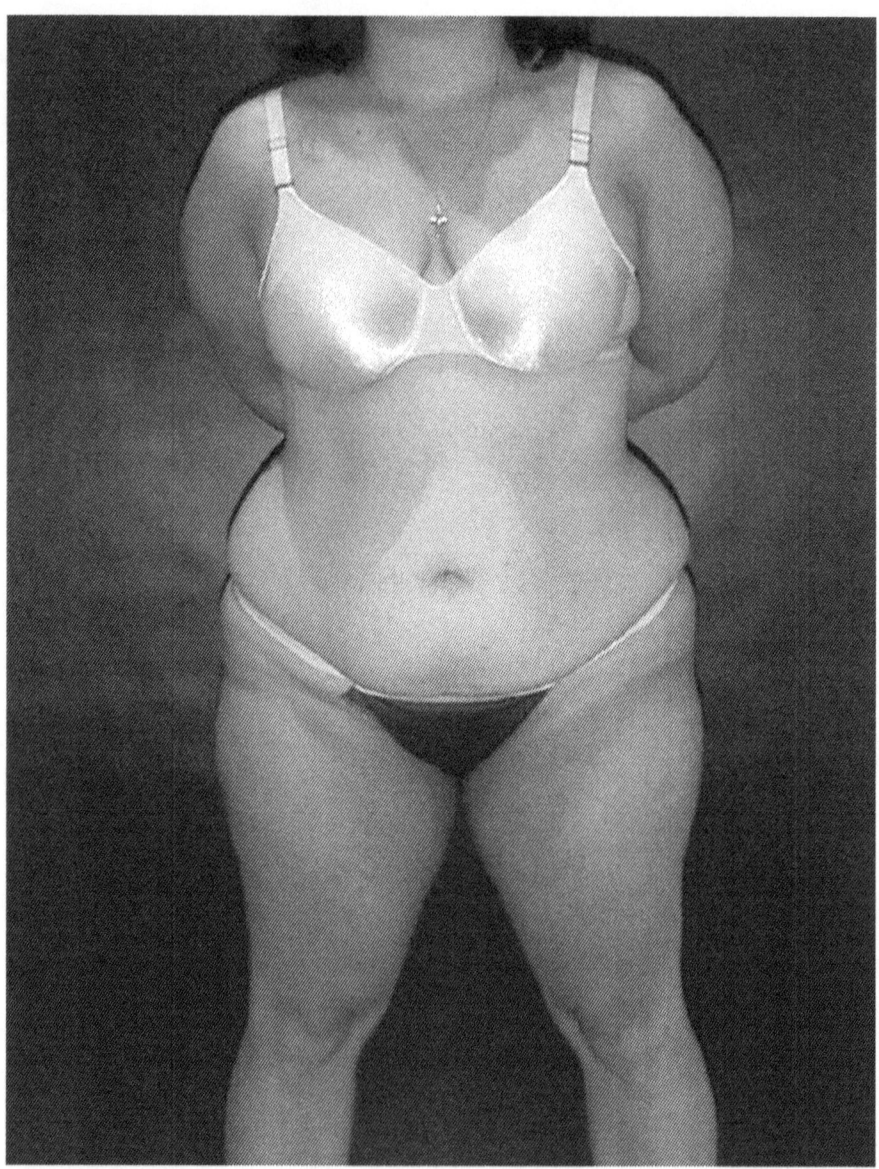

Figure 7.7: Helena came in requesting an abdominoplasty, more commonly referred to as a "tummy tuck". Fortunately she agreed to liposuction and she was able to avoid the extensive scars that go along with the abdominoplasty procedure (see Figures 8.1 and 8.2).

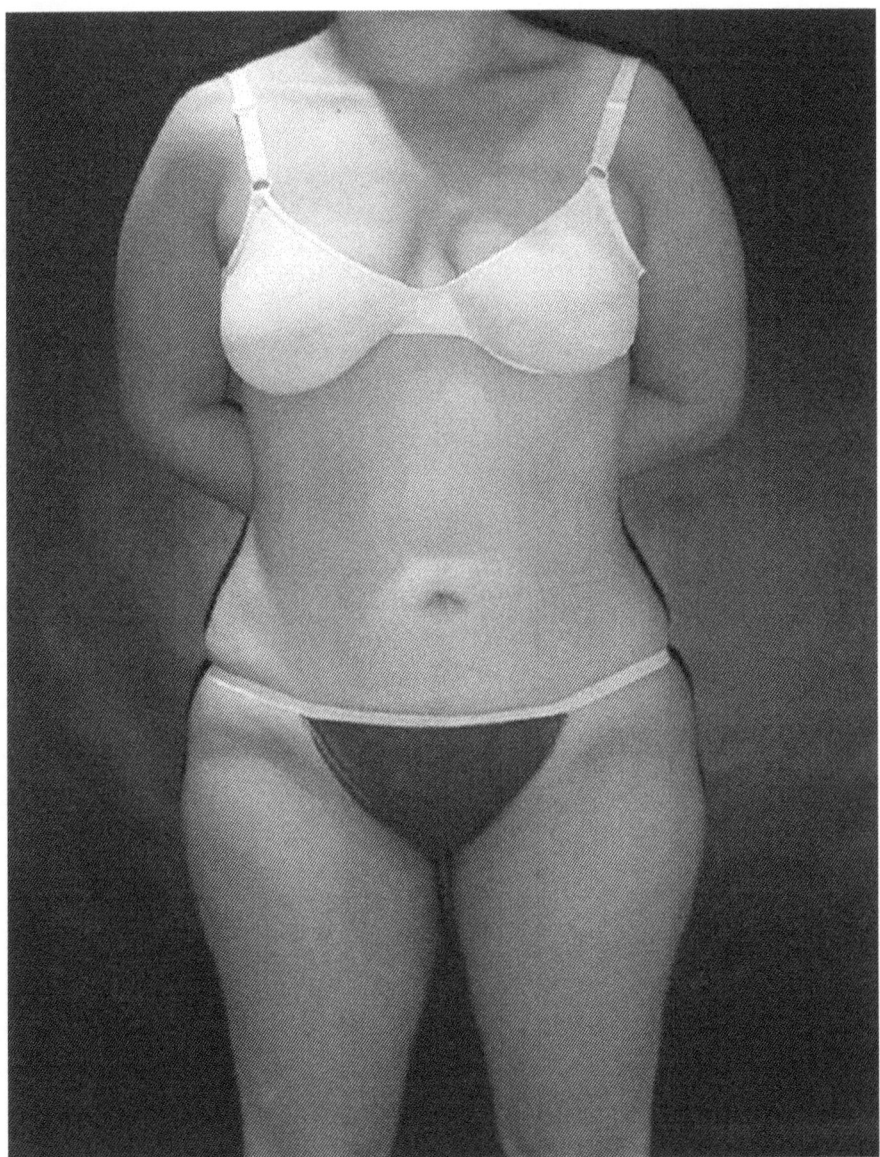

Figure 7.8: Helena was extremely happy with her post-operative results and the fact that there were no visible scars.

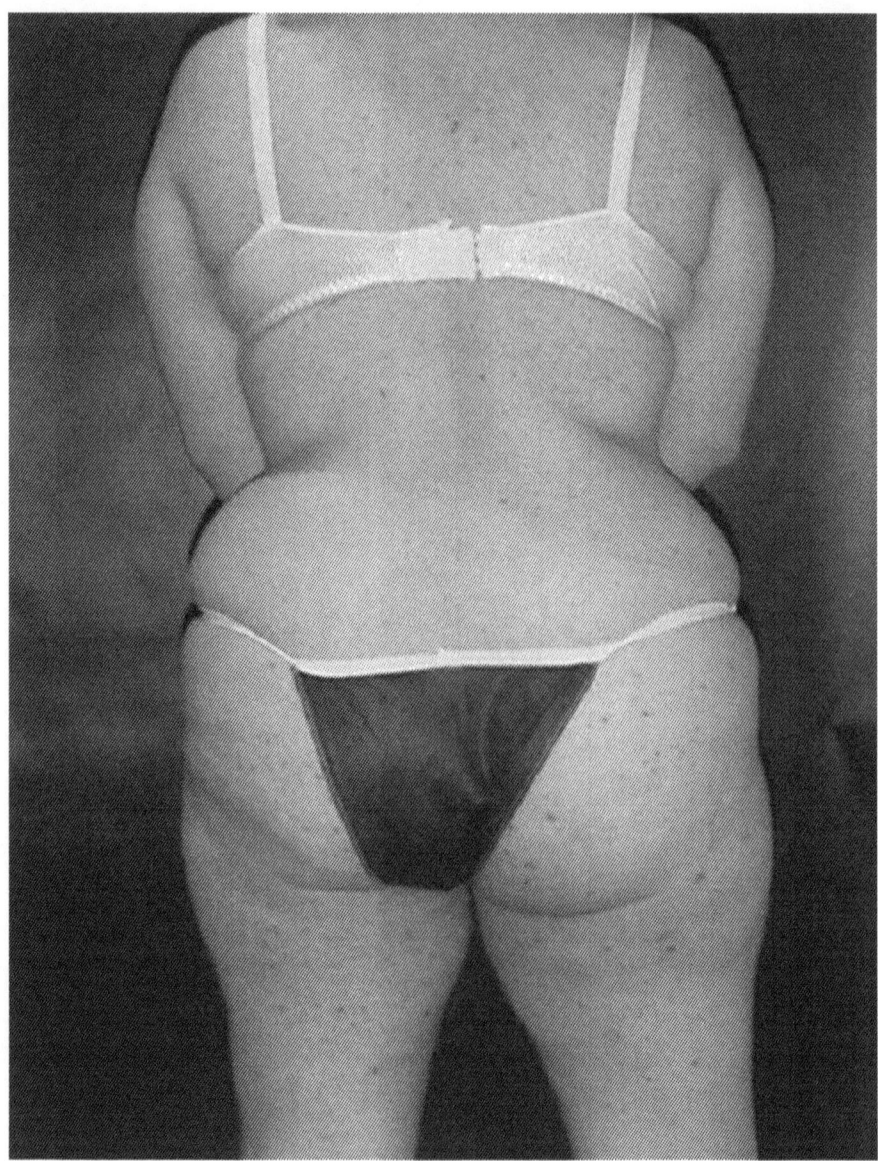

Figure 7.9: Helena in the pre-operative view from behind showing that she needed circumferential liposuction around the waistline.

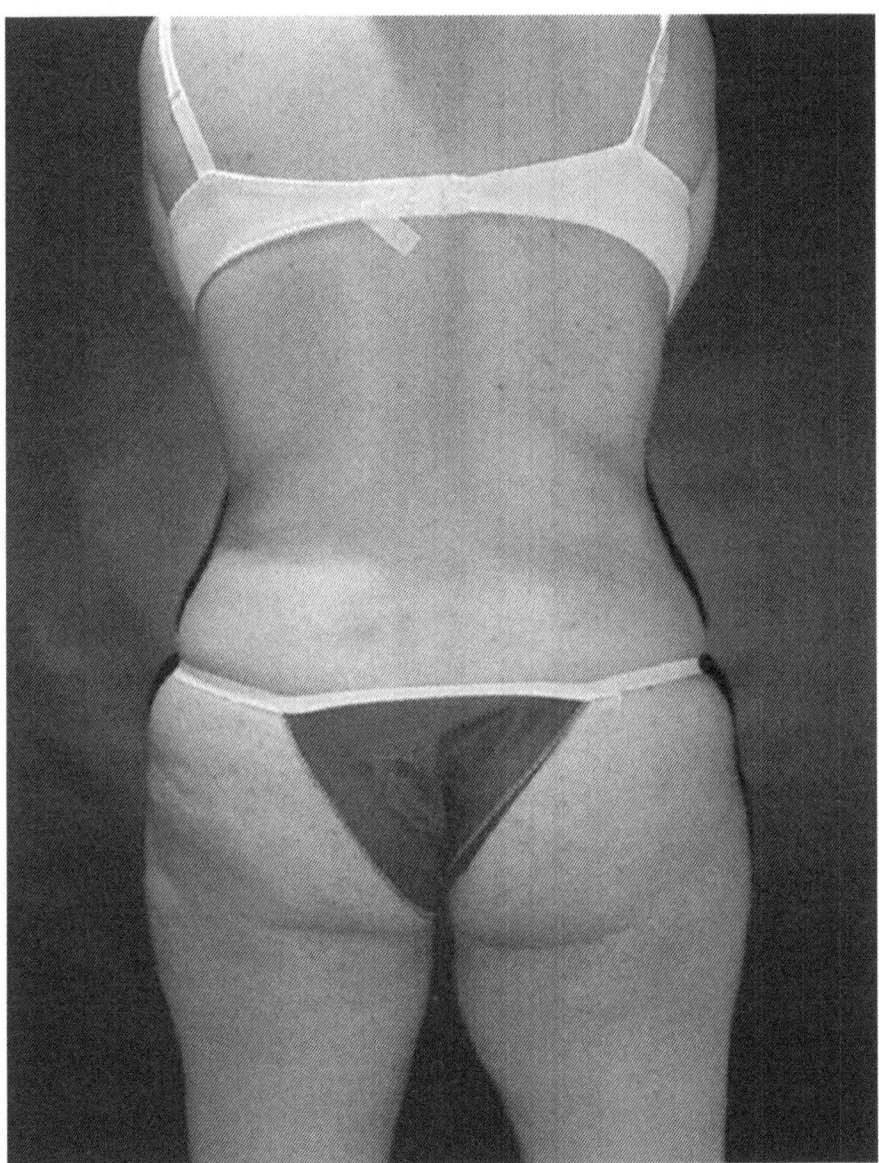

Figure 7.10: Post-operative view of Helena showing the benefits of circum-ferential liposuction.

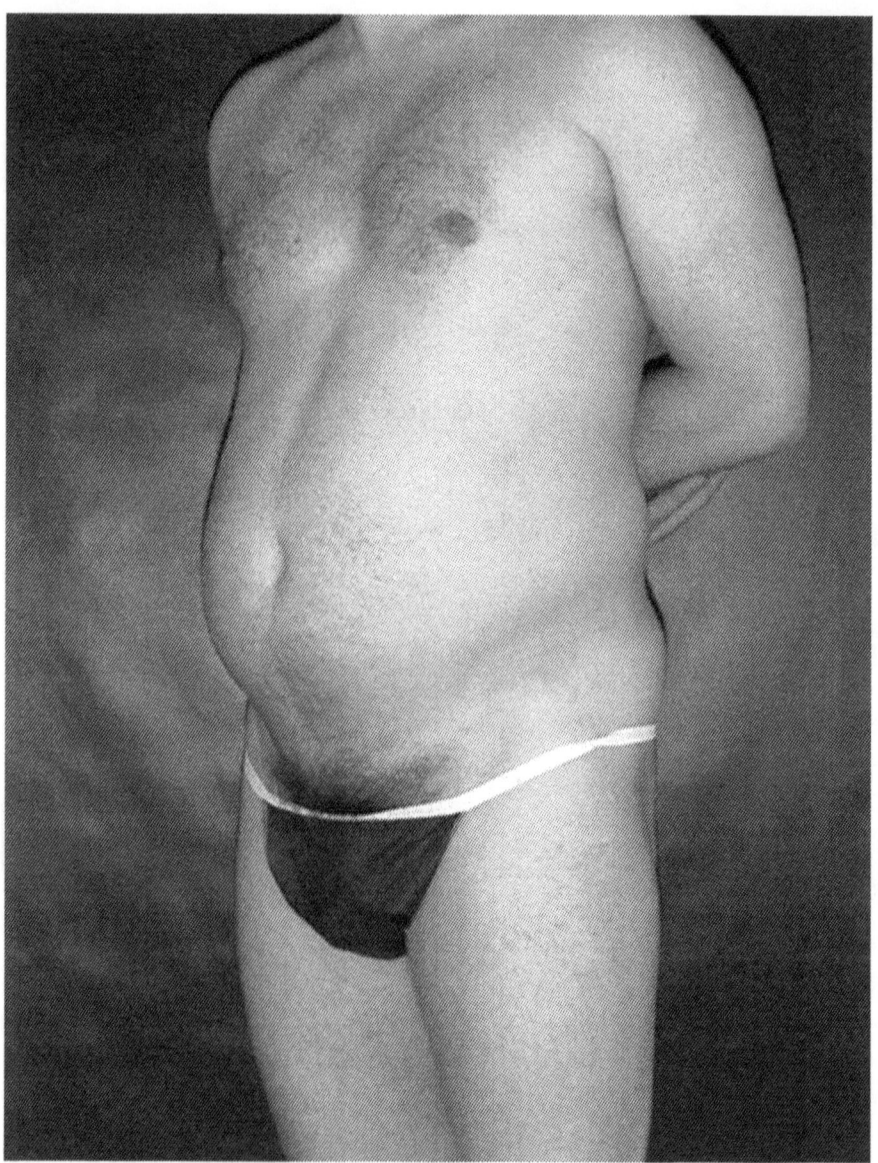

Figure 7.11: Ian, pre-operatively, showing a waistline many inches greater than his chest circumference.

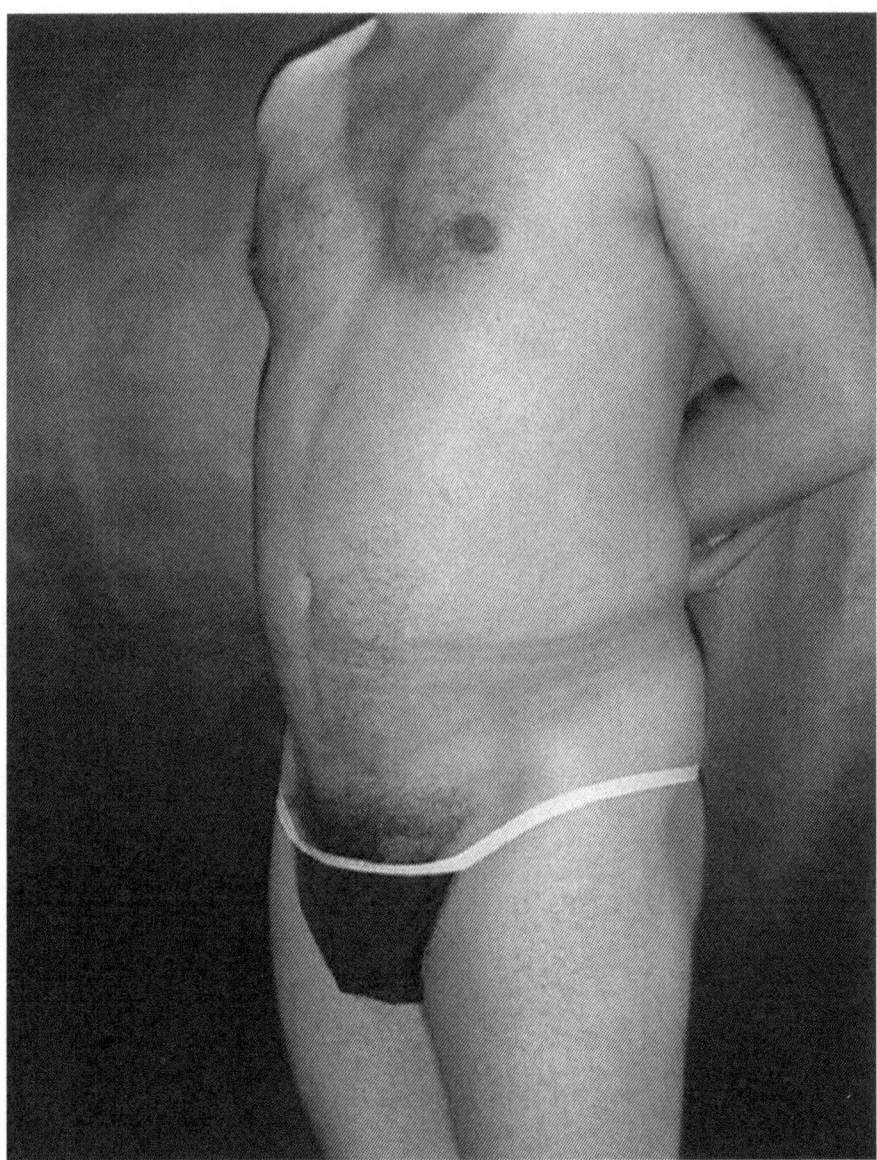

Figure 7.12: Ian, post-operatively, needed to take all his pants to his tailor to have them taken in!

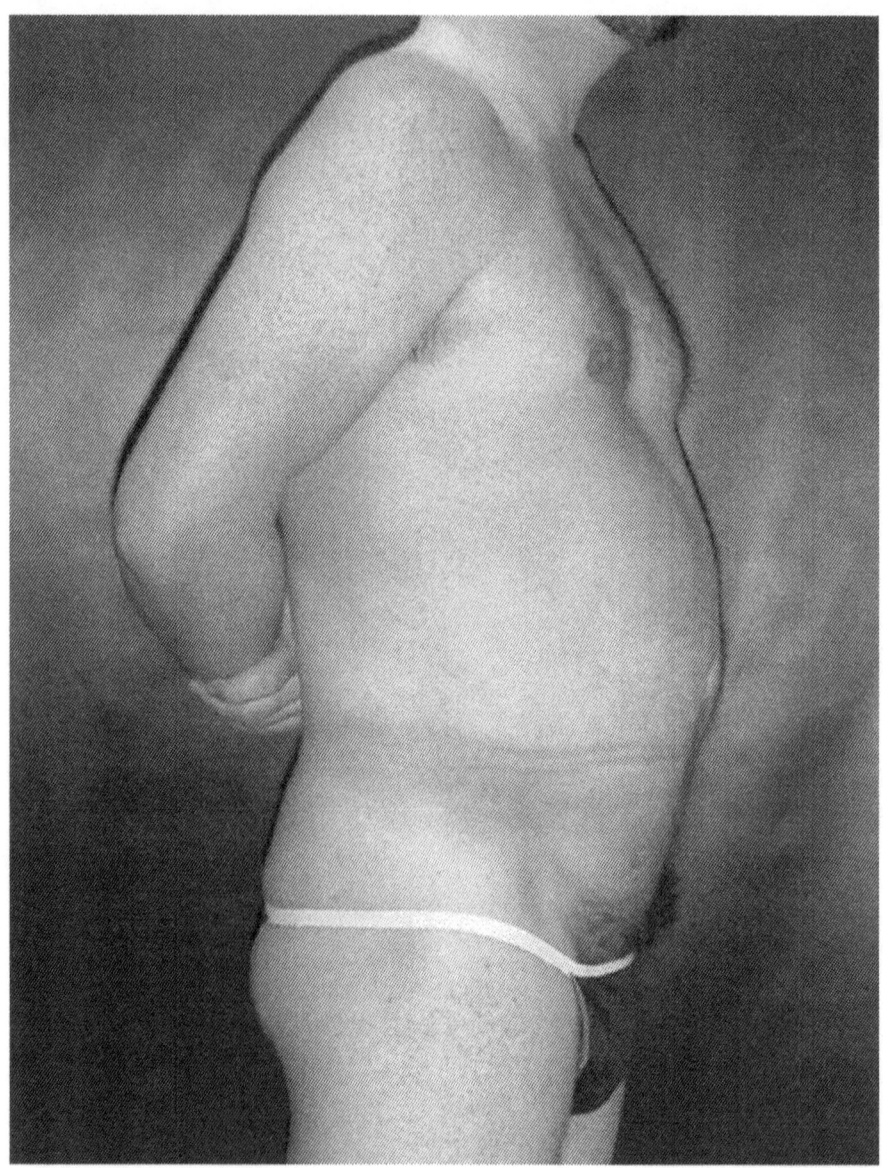

Figure 7.13: Another view of Ian demonstrates that his fat was located above as well as below the belly button.

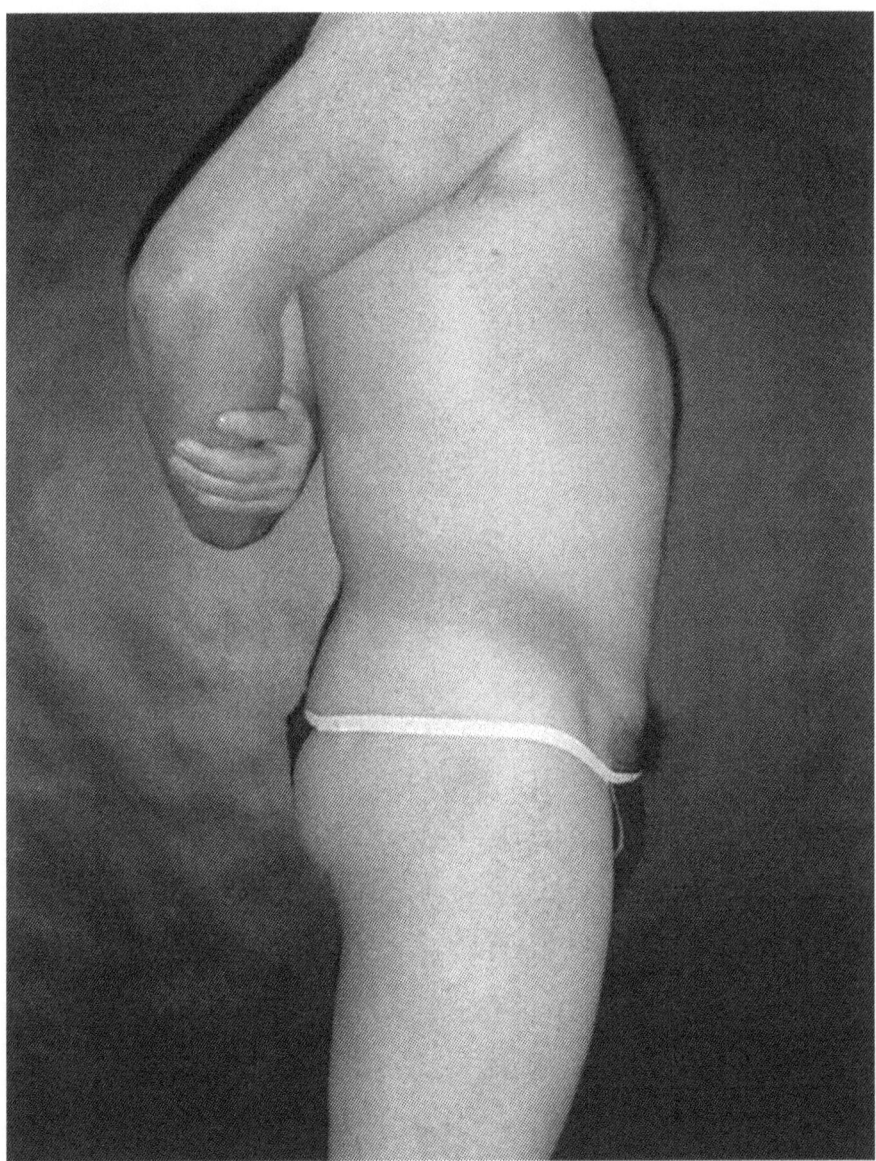

Figure 7.14: Post-operative view of Ian shows that his entire abdomen has been re-contoured with liposuction.

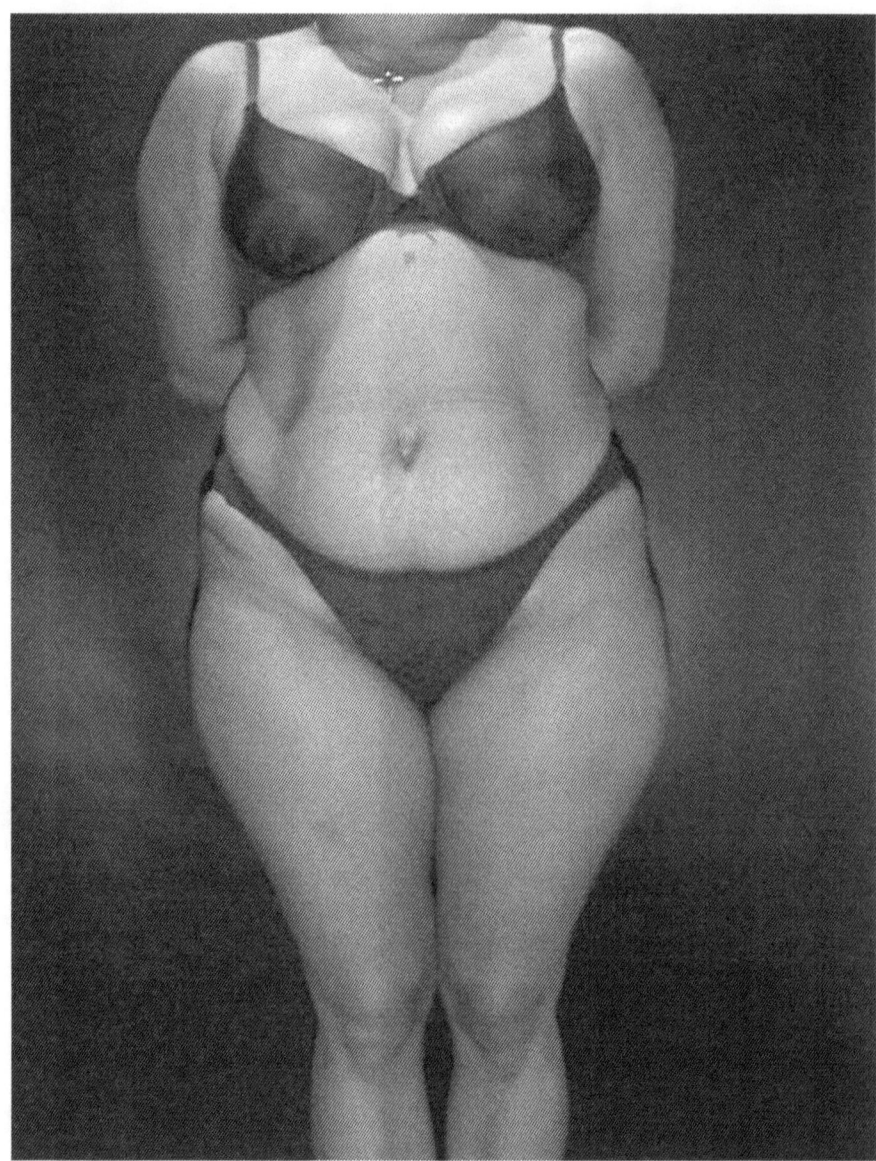

**Figure 7.15: Jaclyn pre-operatively came in for volume liposuction**

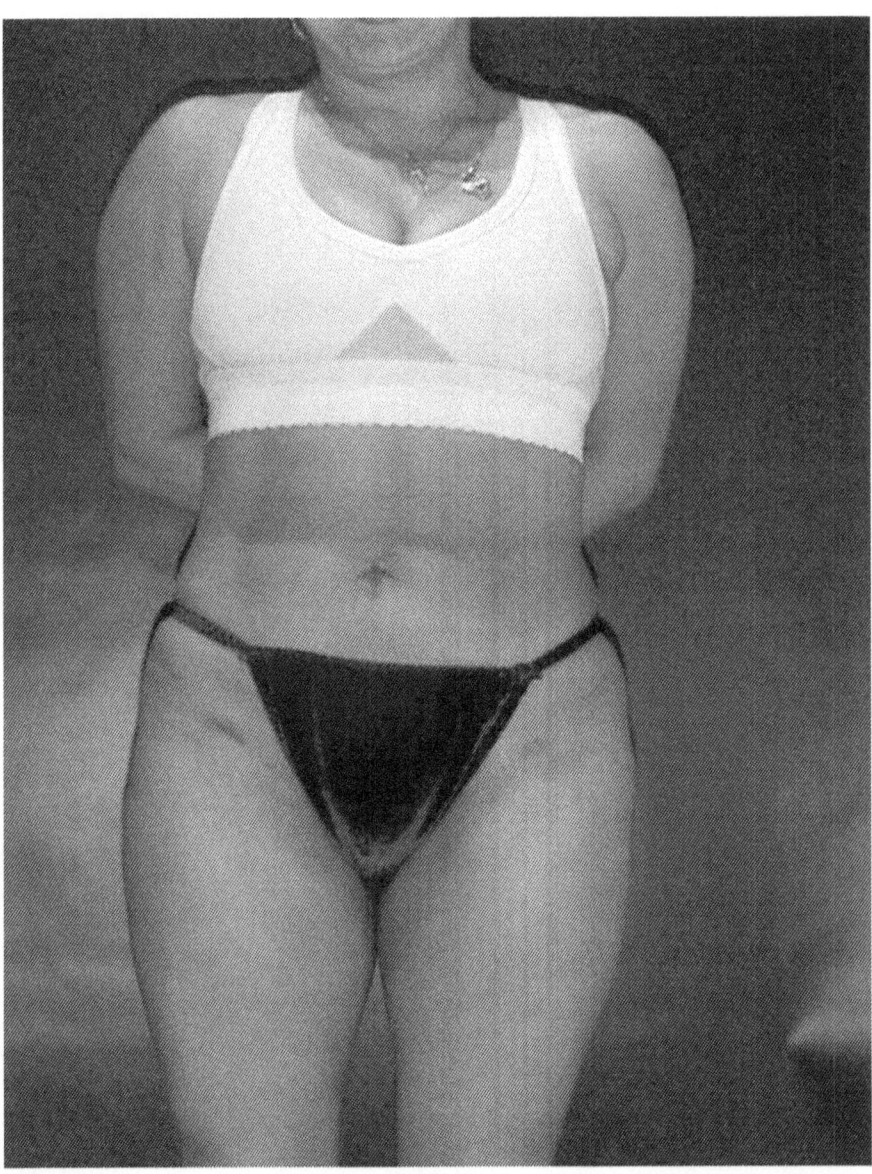

Figure 7.16: A happy Jaclyn showing the results of successful volume liposuction. But now she is also wondering if she could benefit from finesse liposuction.

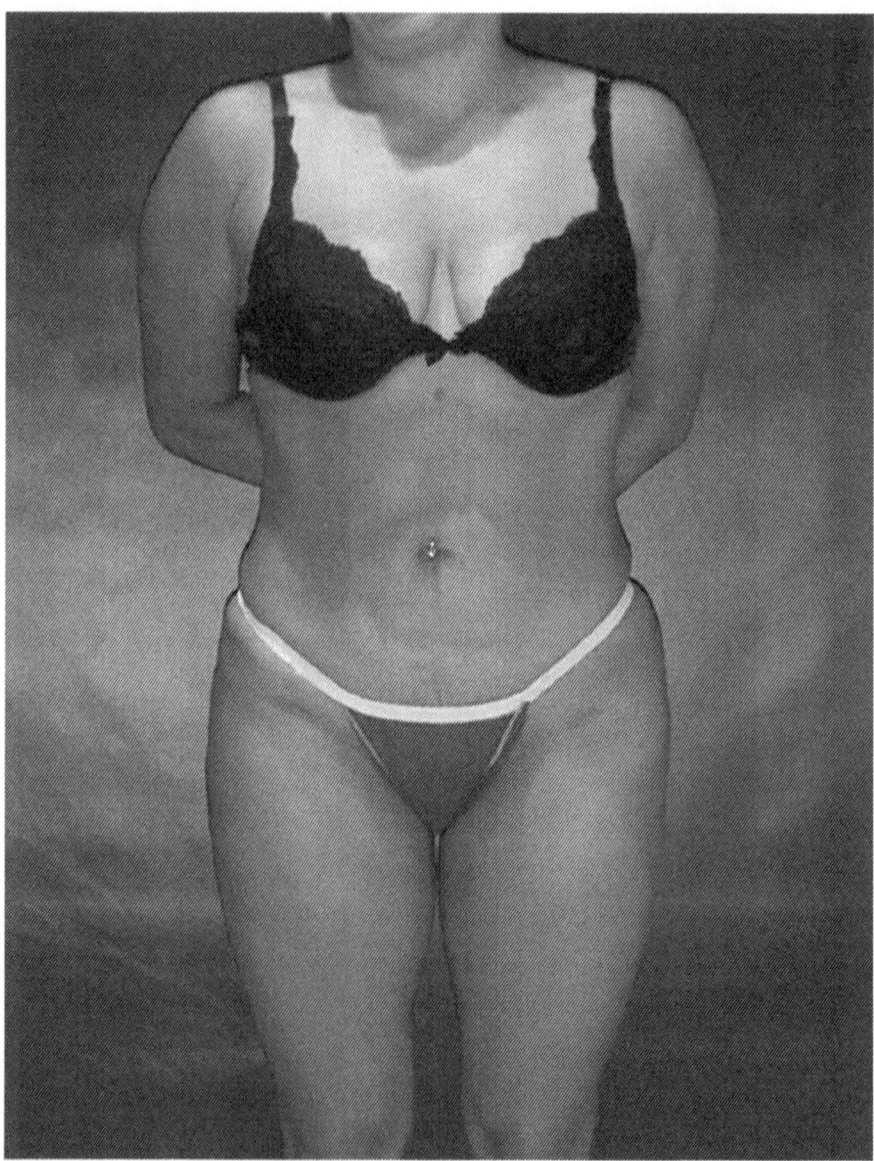

Figure 7.17: Jaclyn following a second liposuction, this time for finesse, showing a dramatic final result.

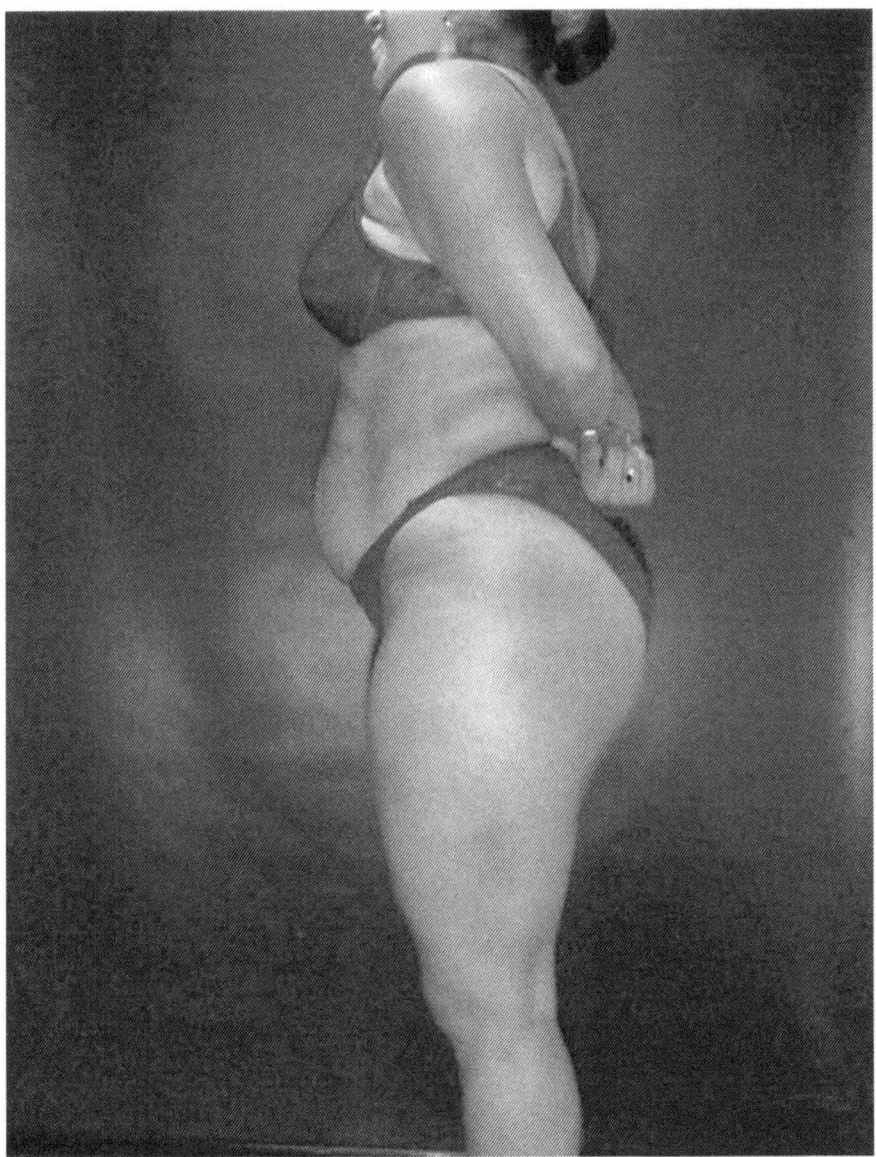

Figure 7.18 Jaclyn before her first liposuction from the side view

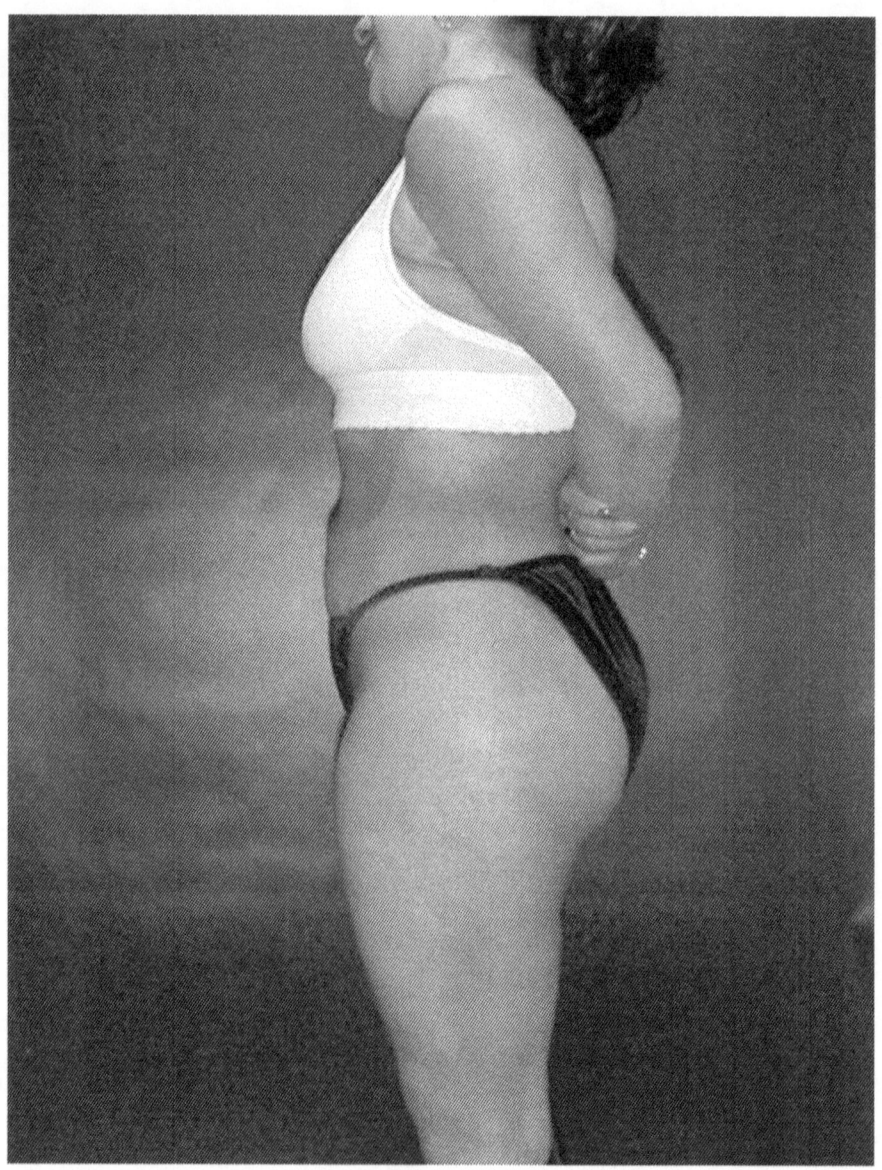

**Figure 7.19: Jaclyn following liposuction for volume reduction.**

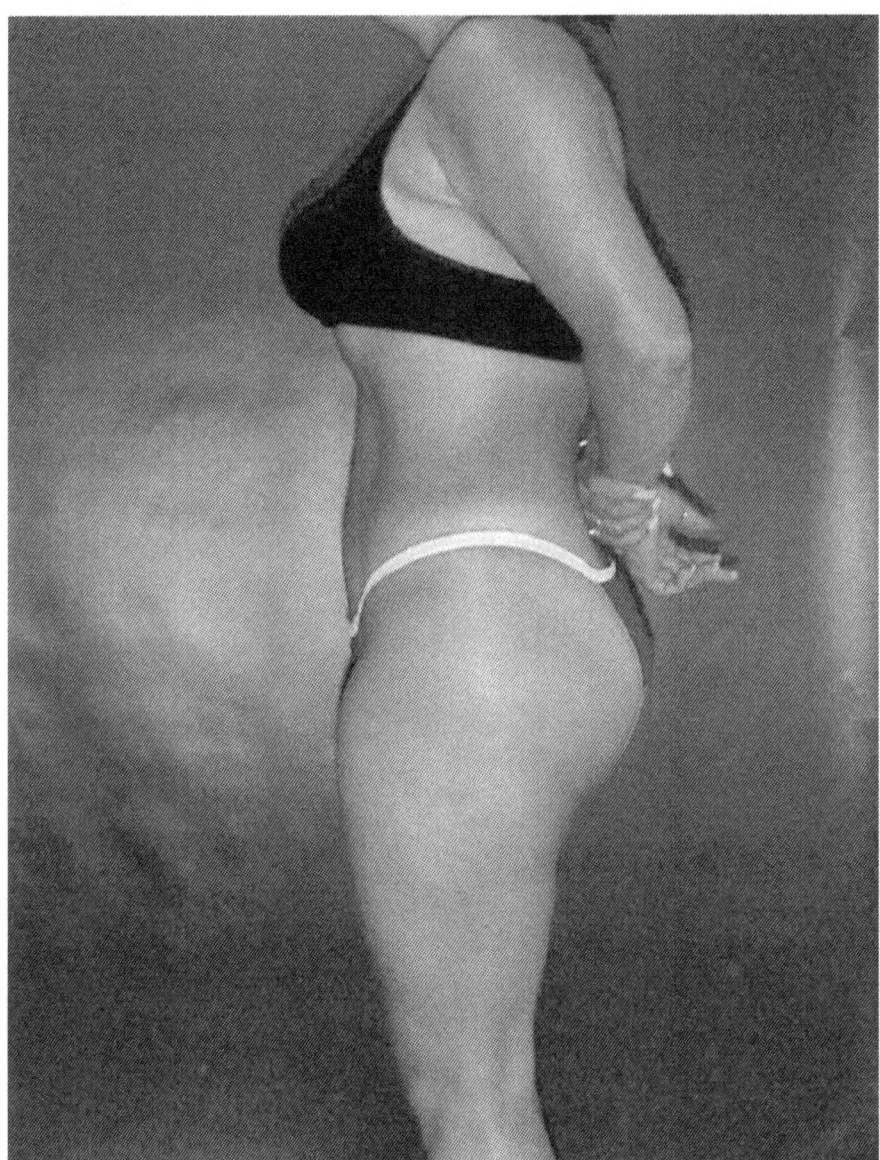

**Figure 7.20 Jaclyn following a second liposuction, this time for finesse.**

# Chapter 8

## Abdominoplasty versus Liposuction

One of the most common questions that patients ask is wether they should have abdominoplasty (tummy tuck) or liposuction. In my view the traditional abdominoplasty procedure is undesirable for most patients. Firstly, it leaves a long scar extending from hip bone to hip bone, and even when the scar heals perfectly I still find the trade-off hard to justify. Also, remember that the popularity of liposuction, since its inception, has been the avoidance of the scars, which revealed that the patient had undergone cosmetic surgery. It is impossible to have a natural looking result, if the tell-tale signs of the surgeon's visitation are there for all to see.

In the traditional abdominoplasty procedure all the skin between the umbilicus above, and the pubic hair below, is removed so that the skin that used to lie above the belly button is stitched to the pubic hair, and the belly button is then pulled through this skin flap and stitched into its new position. Karen (Figs. 8.1-2) is an example of a patient who came to me following traditional abdominoplasty who was dissatisfied with the result of her surgery performed by another surgeon. I examined her carefully and asked her what she was unhappy about. "Well, firstly, I didn't realize that the scar would be so long and the scar is kind of wide. It's not so bad when I have a bikini on but every time I'm with a man, especially for the first time, I'm so embarrassed" she replied, "Is there anything that can be done about it?"

In fact the scar that Karen had was the length of the scar that results from a traditional abdominoplasty. It was actually a pretty good scar because on both sides, by the hip bones where there is little tension on the wound, the scar was excellent. However, as is typical of these incisions, in the middle of the scar where the tension on the wound was maximal the scar had widened. The best that Karen can now hope to achieve would be to revise the scar in this middle portion and hope that it would not spread out again. The length of the scar can't be reduced nor can it be moved to an area where it is less noticeable. Furthermore, there are no lasers, magic potions, or ointments that will make this scar go away.

In fact, even without benefit of Karen's pre-operative pictures, I could pretty confidently say that she had a good to excellent result from the abdominoplasty procedure. The problem lies in the fact that this is the kind of result to be *expected* from the "tummy tuck" procedure. This is the major reason why, in my opinion, as a <u>primary</u> procedure, the traditional abdominoplasty is an outdated procedure. Like many similar post-abdominoplasty patients who come to me for a second opinion I had to tell her the sad truth that she could have been better served with liposuction which would have avoided the "tummy tuck" but that there was little that could be done now that she had the scar. She was quite distraught to hear this but she had not yet finished with her list of complaints about what the abdominoplasty procedure had done to her. Turning around she pointed to the folds in her skin and protuberant fat bulges above her buttocks. "I didn't have these before the surgery," she said, "What happened here?"

Unfortunately, the news was not good, she was not imagining these bulges and skin folds and again even without the benefit of pre-operative pictures I knew she was telling the truth, because this too is a problem with abdominoplasty that not many patients stop to consider before undergoing the procedure. Simply put, like a tight pullover, as the skin at the front of the abdomen is pulled down it bunches up at the back giving rise to these skin folds bulging up with fat within these folds.

Again these new skin folds and fat bulges are not a complication of the abdominoplasty procedure but the expected and inevitable result of pulling the skin down tightly at the front. Fortunately I explained to

Karen we could solve this problem with liposuction. We can suction out the fat and the skin will contract down once the underlying fat is removed. What we have learned from liposuction is that most often the skin is not the problem and it has simply expanded to cover the underlying fat. Once that fat is removed the skin will contract down to cover the new shape and form.

In fact, we should have known this all along. The skin does not do anything by itself! Just as when a woman is pregnant the skin responds by expanding to the underlying expanding womb. After the baby is delivered the skin shrinks rapidly in response to the fact that there is no longer underlying pressure pushing on the skin. As long as the skin has not been so rapidly stretched during pregnancy that the elastic fibers within the skin have been ruptured the skin will shrink. If the fibers were ruptured, by rapid stretching, then they will no longer be able to fulfill their function, and these ruptured fibers will be visible as the stretch marks hated by so many women.

The bad news here is that there is <u>no</u> treatment, which is successful in getting rid of theses stretch marks. I repeat none: no creams, lotions, laser or European spa treatment can replace those ruptured elastic fibers and repair the damage they have wrecked on the skin. Abdominoplasty will excise some of this damaged skin but the trade-off is the long supra-pubic scar. Only in this instance do I consider proposing an abdominoplasty procedure and even then the patient has to consider carefully wether the trade-off is worth it in their mind. In addition the patient has to be reminded that the stretch marks above the umbilicus will not be excised by abdominoplasty and para-doxically as those stretch marks are pulled down they will appear worse! Those stretch marks are in fact further stretched out during abdominoplasty.

From the above remarks you can see that I am no great fan of the abdominoplasty procedure and, when you can achieve equivalent or better results with liposuction of the abdomen, you can understand why. With liposuction you can also achieve things such as circumfer-ential liposuction around the waist, which simply cannot be achieved with abdominoplasty. In addition, there are no visible scars to give away the fact that the patient has undergone surgery. The final factor that argues in favor of liposuction is that even in the small proportion of patients in whom the skin does not shrink completely they can still undergo abdominoplasty. In my experience this is very rarely required but at least that option is still there.

Most commonly the skin responds extremely well to liposuction and rapidly shrinks to conform to the reduced waist size. In fact, there is an additional reason as to why this happens. It is not simply that the skin is conforming to the reduced waist size, but, in fact, during liposuction, everywhere the liposuction cannula is going in the subcutaneous fat it is causing some micro-scarring and this scar is also causing the skin to contract. This is one of the few instances in plastic surgery that I can think of where scar contracture is helping to enhance the result as opposed to the usual situation, where scar contracture is the enemy. Remember that the tiny skin puncture wounds where the cannula was introduced are simply incision sites, and the scar I am referring to is actually the entire subcutaneous area where the cannula went. Post-operatively, like any scar, this scar will feel hard to the touch as you run your hand over the liposuctioned areas and over time, as the scar softens and matures, the normal softness returns. Most patients are pleased to have the normal softness of their body back, although this is also the end point of the skin shrinkage and the patient has gained the maximum benefit to be achieved from the liposuction. This usually happens about three months after the surgery.

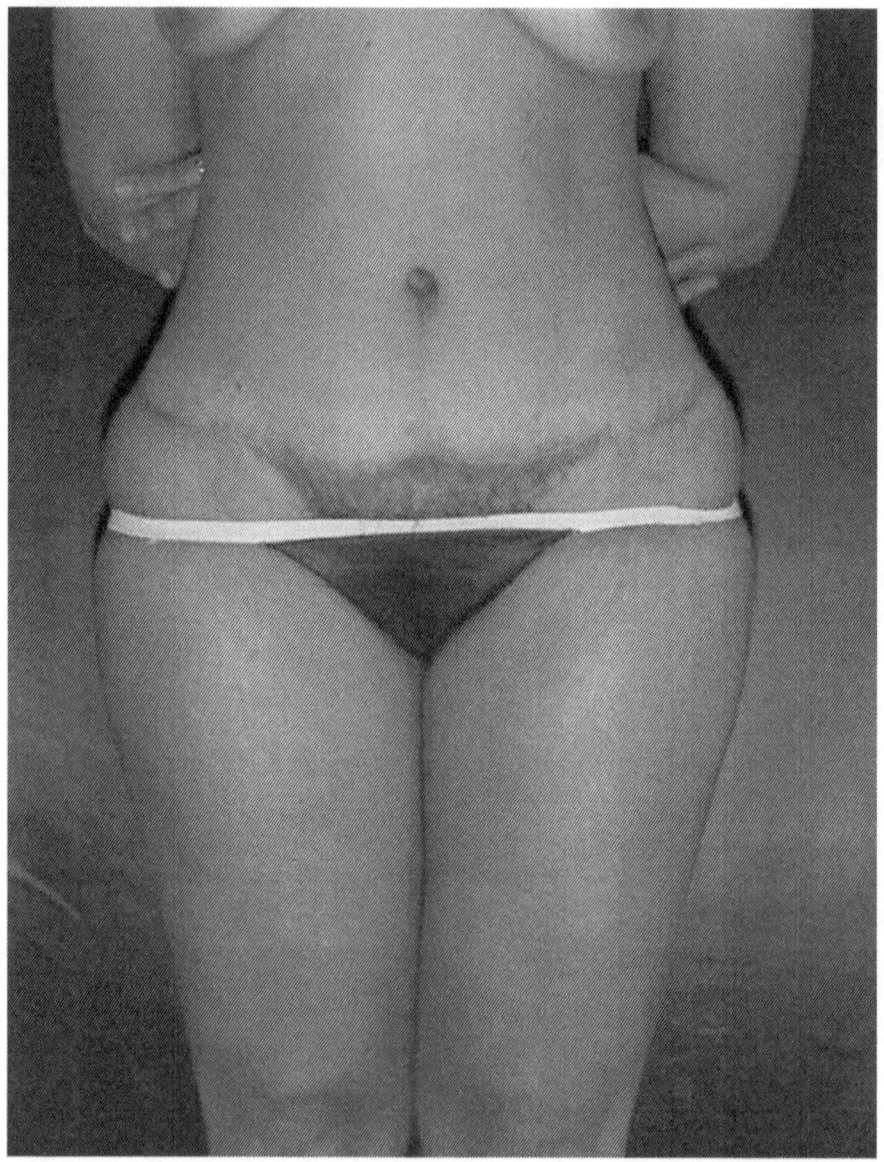

Figure 8.1: Karen had abdominoplasty, by another surgeon, and is now unhappy with the scar for which unfortunately there is little that can be done. She would have been better served by agreeing to volume liposuction, see Figures 7.7-10.

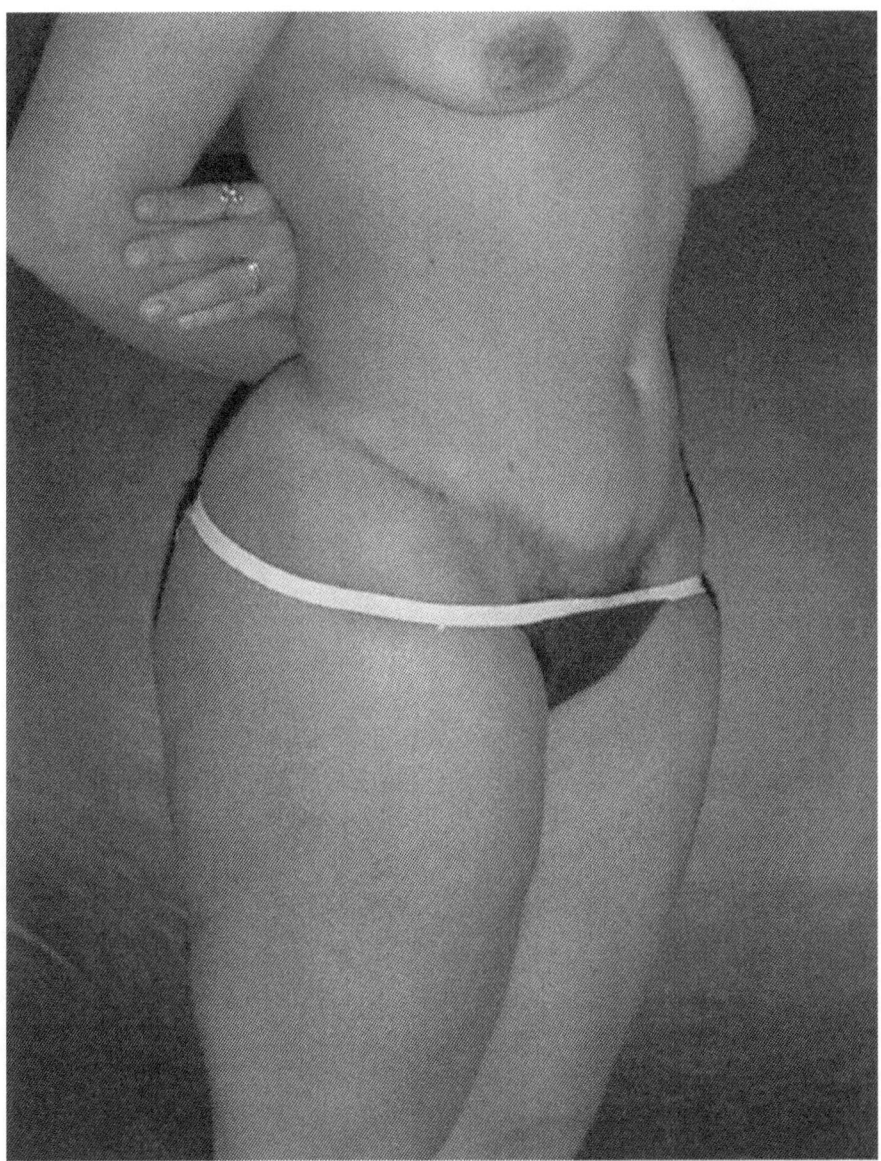

Figure 8.2: Karen's scar is *not* a complication but the kind of result to be *expected* from an abdominoplasty procedure (tummy tuck).

# Chapter 9

## Breast Reduction Surgery using Liposuction

Gynecomastia is the medical term for enlarged breasts in male patients and this can be a very distressing condition leading the patient to seek medical consultation. Very rarely there can be a medical reason as to why the patient's breasts have enlarged but most commonly there is no reason why this should have happened and it is left to explain to the patient that all needs to be done is to simply reduce the size of the breasts.

Prior to the introduction of liposuction this would entail a surgical operation in which the excess skin and breast tissue were excised and the remaining tissue was tailored to achieve the appearance of a normal breast. This inevitably involved scars wherever the skin was being cut. Often the trade-off, a smaller chest with scars, for the original gynecomastia, was not one the patient, or the surgeon, was happy with. The avoidance of these scars was the motivating force to consider liposuctioning of the male breast.

The breast, in both male and female patients, is predominantly fatty tissue interspersed throughout the breast lobules and ducts, which are more fibrous and have a different consistency than fat. Initial attempts to liposuction the male breast were not terribly successful because it was difficult to remove the fat as it was encased within these fibrous ducts and lobules and the cannulae simply could not get to all the fat because of the barrier that this fibrous tissue presented. This limitation was overcome with the introduction of ultrasonic liposuction where the energy from the probe was able to emulsify the fat, even through the ductal tissue in which it was encased, and then the emulsified fat could be removed.

Correction of gynecomastia is one of the conditions in which ultrasonic liposuction really comes into its own and most surgeons agree that satisfactory results can be achieved only by ultrasonic liposuction. If you suffer from gynecomastia, I can tell you with confidence that no amount of exercising of your chest muscles will reduce the size of your enlarged breasts. Exercising the pectoral muscles, especially with intensive weight training, will definitely increase the size of the pectoral muscles but will do nothing directly to the overlying breast tissue, either to increase or decrease the size of the breasts. Only by directly working on the breast tissue with ultrasonic liposuction can you change its shape.

Similarly for women, exercising the pectoral muscles will not increase or decrease the size of their breasts! Only by sufficient exercise to reduce the total body fat content will the female breast begin to decrease in size but that usually requires a level of intensive training that only professional female bodybuilders can achieve so don't worry if you are exercising an hour a day five days a week. It will make no difference to the size of your breasts. They respond only to hormonal changes and weight gain or loss.

The success of breast reduction utilizing liposuction in the male patients has led some surgeons to try liposuction of the female breast for breast reduction. There has been significant success in doing so and patients who have suffered from back and shoulder pains due to the weight of their large breasts have been delighted to be able to reduce the size of their breasts without the scars associated with traditional breast reduction procedures. However other surgeons, including myself, have been slow to utilize this new use for liposuction for the following reason. One female in eleven in the United States will develop breast cancer in her lifetime. Naturally, if the patient who had liposuction of the breast to reduce the breast size were to develop breast cancer she might blame it on the surgery. While there is no evidence that there is any correlation between breast reduction surgery and the incidence of breast cancer many surgeons have opted to wait until more information is available. In any case if your surgeon does offer this procedure then he will ask you to sign a special consent form for liposuction reduction of the breast. However, at this point in time, I believe that liposuction is going to play an important role in breast reduction surgery for females also and I have begun to offer this procedure to my patients.

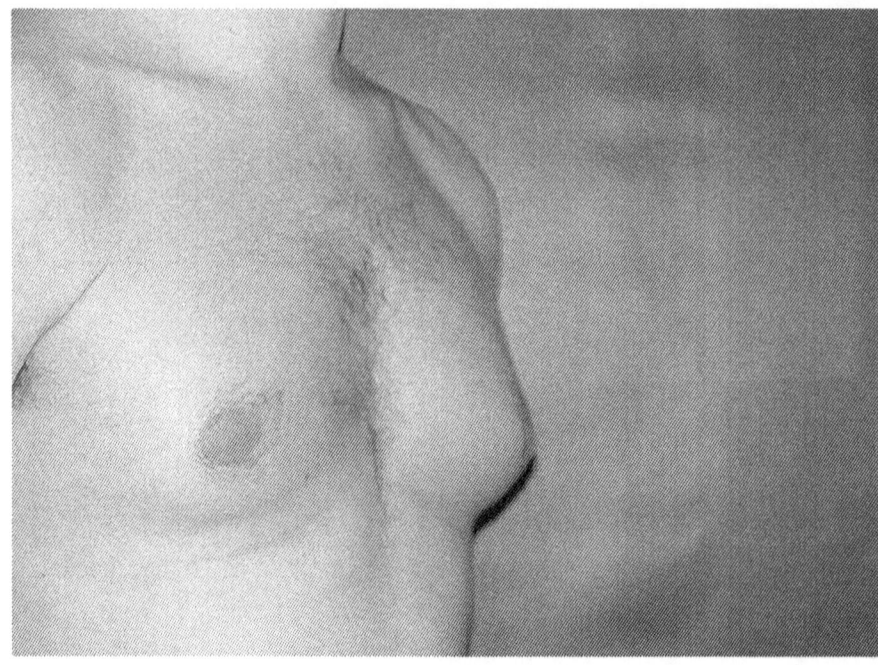

Figure 9.1 Liam, has been bothered by his gynecomastia for many years prior to seeking surgery.

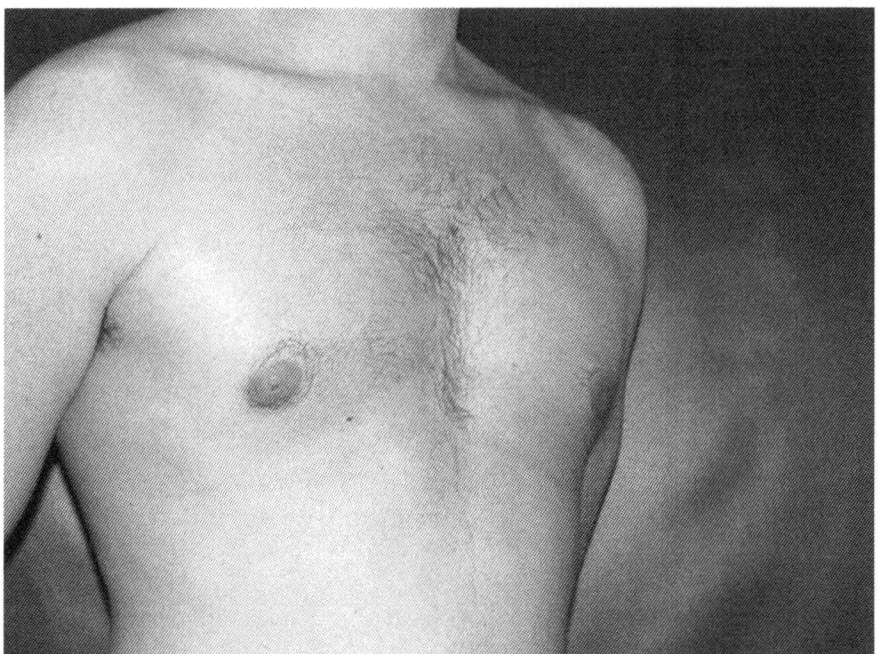

Figure 9.2: Liam, following ultrasonic liposuction to correct his gynecomastia, shows a much more masculine contour.

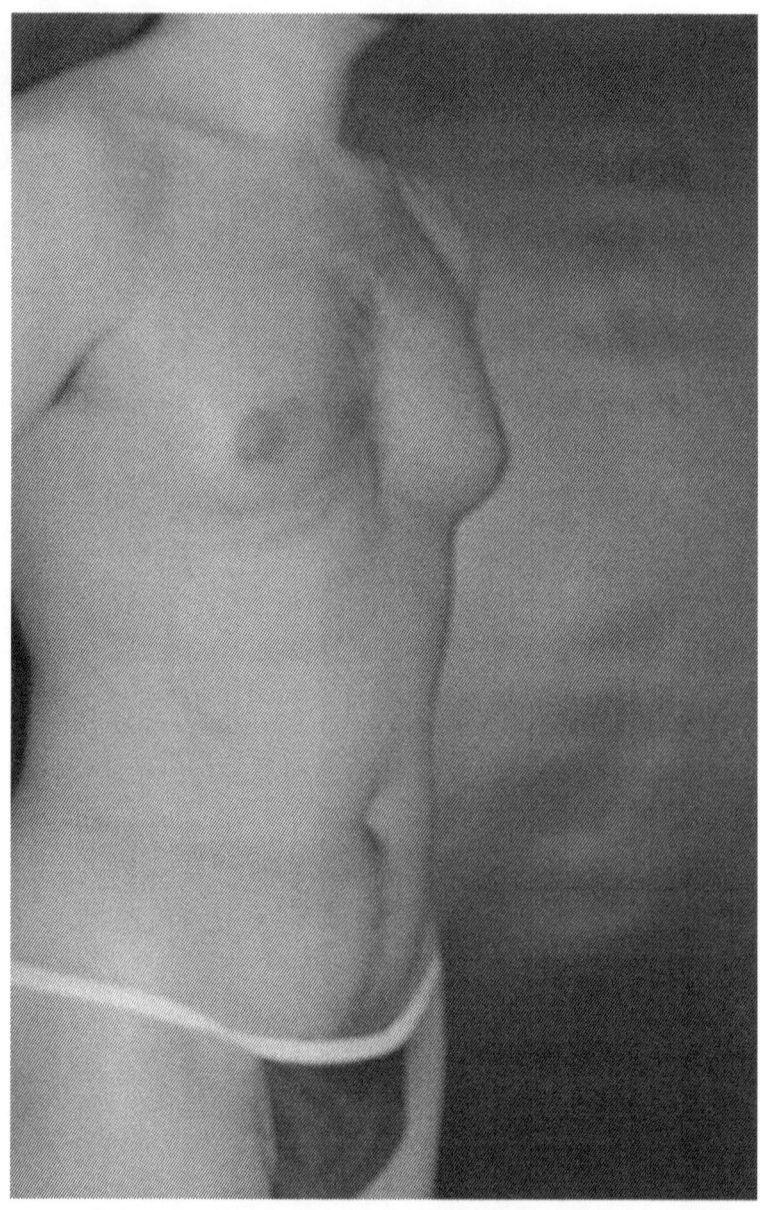

Figure 9.3: Full-length picture of Liam pre-operatively showing the disproportion resulting from enlarged breasts.

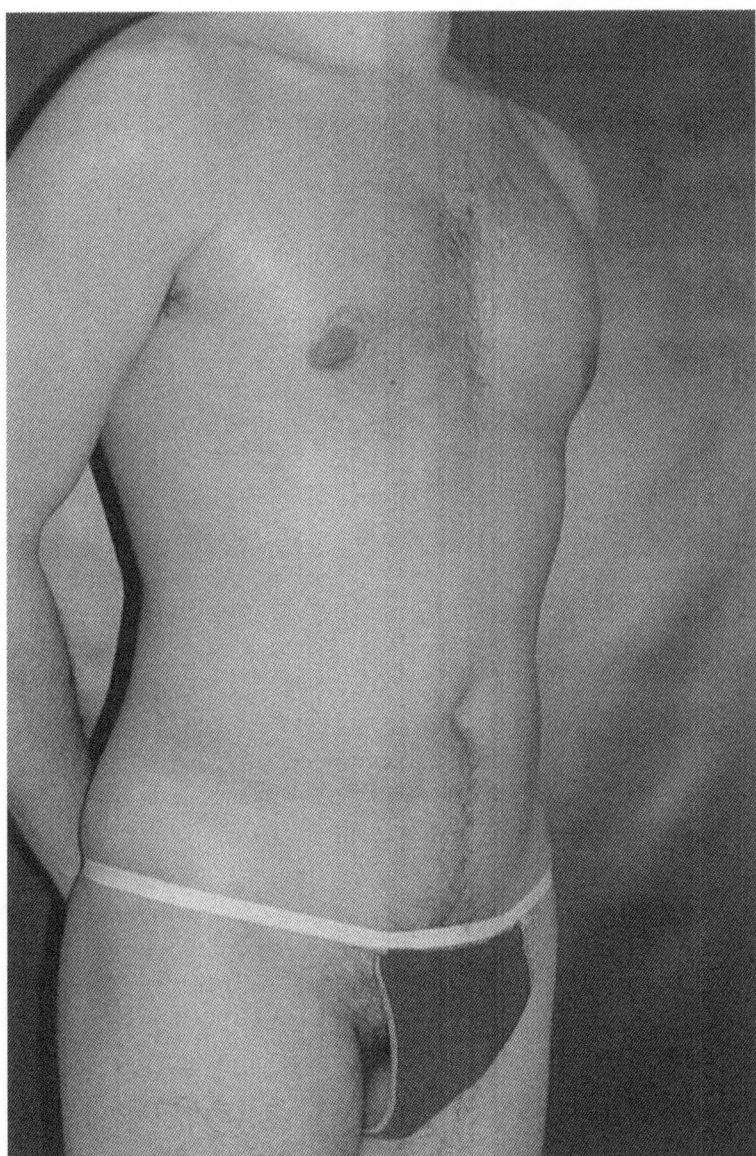

Figure 9.4: Liam's post-operative picture shows the definition that ultrasonic liposuction achieved. Liam, like many patients, had tried to achieve this change unsuccessfully for many years with diet and exercise.

# Chapter 10

## How much will Liposuction cost?

In New York City, where I practice, costs are just a little bit higher than the rest of the country so the fees quoted here may not be representative of the rest of the country. However, wherever you are in the country there are three main costs associated with liposuction surgery. Firstly, is the fee to be paid to the anesthesiologist. This typically is a straight forward hourly rate, presently about $350 per hour, regardless of wether you have selected general anesthesia, "twilight anesthesia," or local standby. There may be some additional charges for medications used, but the thing that patients have to understand is that once they have selected a date for surgery the anesthesiologist has to be paid for his time. Once he has accepted your assignment he cannot be in any other place at that time. In fact as anesthesiologists are fond of quoting, "You only pay for my time. The training, expertise, and caring that I bring to you during the critical hours during and after surgery you get for free. But for my time I have to be reimbursed."

The second cost is a facility fee for wherever the surgery is to be performed. This may be the hospital, a freestanding surgery center or the plastic surgeon's office. There are certain minimum costs for equipping and maintaining an operating room and the skilled personnel to run it and in New York in a private office that runs about $500 per hour. It will cost more than that in a freestanding surgical center, and higher still in a hospital.

Most patient's prefer to have surgery in the doctor's office, not simply because it costs less, but because of the privacy factor. After finishing training in 1989 I didn't have facilities in my office to perform surgery and I was doing all my surgery at the hospital. One of my patients after the surgery told me, "Doctor, you did a really nice job and I'm very pleased with the results, but honestly I would never go through with it again". I asked her why. "Well when I went to the hospital the admitting clerk asked me what I was there for, and, really, I felt that it was none of his business. Then the IV technician who drew my blood asked me about the surgery, the orderly who wheeled me to the operating room asked me, and the girl in day surgery was curious as to wether I really needed the surgery. It just went on and on. I really was nervous enough already on the morning of surgery, and I just didn't need everyone inquiring into my business at that point". Needless to say, I decided pretty rapidly after that I should find office facilities where I could operate on my patients in privacy.

The third fee is what the surgeon actually charges for the surgery and while the costs for the anesthesiologist and facility fee are relatively constant the surgical fee will vary with the length of time the surgeon has been in practice, his expertise in that particular field, and the technical difficulty of the surgery. Believe me, liposuctioning fat out of the face is much more technically demanding than taking fat out of the abdomen. The demand for the surgeon's services, and the length of time the proposed surgery will take and the level of postoperative aftercare anticipated all play a part in the level of fee quoted. It really is very difficult to quote a surgical fee without examining the patient but it can be as little as $1500 for a finesse liposuction, (think about the size of a grapefruit), to $5000 for a large volume liposuction, (think about two two-liter milk cartons). However even a finesse liposuction in the area of the neck and face will run to the higher end of this schedule because of the technical demands of working in this area.

These are the three primary costs associated with liposuction, but there may also be some other minor charges for blood work and other pre-operative tests if required, pre and post-operative photographs and compression garments.

As a general rule, all the fees are required to be paid at the time a surgery date is scheduled. Also the fees for the anesthesiologist and the facility are not refundable because that time, once blocked off, cannot be rescheduled if, for any reason, the patient decides to cancel the surgery. Similarly, most surgeons will charge a cancellation fee although this is usually only 50% of the fee that was charged.

Cosmetic surgery, of course, is not covered by health insurance and these costs are all out-of-pocket expenses to the patient. While for many patients this is not a problem, for others these expenditures can be a stretch on their budget. To serve these patients, a whole host of financing companies have sprung up to allow patients to spread the cost of the surgery over a three or five year term. Some of these companies even advertise directly to the public with headlines like "You too can have a new body through liposuction for as little as $99 a month!"

Patients simply have to remember that these finance companies are providing unsecured loans and that the interest rates on these loans can be well over 18%. In addition to that, they may charge a fee to the surgeon's office and while most surgeons' fees already reflect the 2% they pay to Visa or American Express when they accept those credit cards these finance companies may be charging up to 10% and the surgeon's office will simply increase the fees correspondingly to cover this cost.

What this all really means is that cosmetic surgery is still a luxury for most people and while attempts to democratize its availability and bring it within reach of people of average financial means are commendable they come with a cost that the patient should be aware of. Nevertheless, despite the cost, more than 250,000 Americans a year are having liposuction. This probably translates into one adult American in 500 undergoing this procedure each year, so I can only believe, all these patients believe the cost are worth the benefits.

# Chapter 11

## Choosing a Surgeon for your Liposuction

This is the most significant choice you will make regarding your surgery and one of the most confusing for patients. The confusion arises from the number of doctors going around calling themselves plastic or cosmetic surgeons, when they simply do not have the requisite training, experience or credentials to do so.

The gold standard is a physician who has completed a residency in Plastic and Reconstructive Surgery that was approved by the American Board of Plastic Surgery. Following this residency, he or she is eligible to sit the two-part examination that leads to the term Board Certified. In the interim the young doctor can obtain privileges at a hospital, commence private practice and is commonly noted to be Board Eligible. This signifies that he has completed the requisite training, but has not yet completed and passed the examinations set by the American Board of Plastic Surgery. For their own internal reasons the term "Board Certified", while in widespread usage, is not officially sanctioned by the American Board of Plastic Surgery and the correct term would be "Baldev S Sandhu M.D., Diplomate American Board of Plastic Surgery"—which is quite a mouthful.

To become a Diplomate the young plastic surgeon has to first pass a written examination in the Principles and Practice of Plastic Surgery, and then, be subjected to an all day oral examination, which is based upon cases selected from an actual audit of the young surgeon's practice and also cases assembled by the Board Examiners. Although I keep saying the young plastic surgeon, in reality, because, of the extended training these physicians have undergone, very few of them are under thirty-four years of age by the time they come to take this second examination. Passing this exam, which is a major milestone, is the basis of the term Board Certified and allows the happy surgeon to apply for membership in the American Society of Plastic Surgeons, which is the oldest association of Plastic Surgeons in the United States and dates back to 1931. The Society maintains a toll-free number (888-4 PLASTIC), which you can call and check to see if a Plastic Surgeon you are interested in is a member or not. Full or active membership in this society automatically means that the surgeon also has been certified by the American Board of Plastic Surgery.

Now this may not seem important, but it is important for you, as a patient, to know the nuances of these terms and why they are important. The American Board of Plastic Surgery, while a private incorporated company with an elected Board of Directors, is actually a quasi-governmental organization. It is responsible to the Committee on Graduate Medical Education, which governs all the different Boards including Internal Medicine, General Surgery, and Pediatrics etc.

All these Boards that have standing with the Committee on Graduate Medical Education are also responsible for the inspection of the training programs in their specialty at the various hospitals and University Medical Centers around the country. Failure to meet their standards will result in de-certification of a training program no matter how prestigious or important the university or medical center. This is the core authority of these Boards that are recognized by the Committee on Graduate Medical Education.

However, there are some Boards which have been organized privately that do not have standing with the Committee on Graduate Medical Education and they too have been handing out diplomas and of course their members too are "Board-Certified". The question to ask really is Board Certified in what and by whom. As I noted earlier the gold standard is certification by the American Board of Plastic Surgery and membership in the American Society of Plastic Surgeons

However, there is absolutely nothing in the law to stop someone, even you, from setting up, let us say for example, the American Board of Liposuction Surgeons. You too could then, at your discretion, certify surgeons who could quite honestly then say that they were "Board-Certified". If someone else has already had the foresight to set up the American Board of Liposuction Surgeons you could perhaps expand your horizons and organize the International Board of Liposuction Surgeons or some other such organization with Board in its title.

While the American Board of Plastic Surgery has only four thousand or so Diplomates, there are many more physicians than that who are holding themselves out to be "Board Certified" and qualified to practice cosmetic surgery and liposuction therefore it behooves you to ask, "Board certified by whom and in what?".

One of the most common problems, in fact are physicians who are Board Certified, but practicing outside the scope of their speciality. For example, in New York City, I know of doctors who are Board Certified by the American Board of Obstetrics and Gynecology who are performing liposuction even though their Board clearly says that is outside the scope of their certification. Similarly there are Diplomates of the American Board of Oral Surgery and Otolaryngology who are performing breast augmentation and while both Boards say that is outside the area of their certification there is nothing to stop these physicians from doing so or performing liposuction of the abdomen or hips.

While these doctors may be excellent physicians and even have undertaken additional training in cosmetic surgery they are still not Board Certified by the American Board of Plastic Surgery because they have not undertaken a training program reviewed and approved by that Board

Every so often, there is some scandal in the newspapers when it is discovered that some physician who was practicing cosmetic surgery outside the scope of his or her certification ran into problems that he or she could not properly manage. When the patient suffers harm in such a case questions are asked about how such an incident could happen. The answer is related to the fragmented nature of physician regulation. For instance, a physician like myself has to be licensed by the State in which they practice. The license to practice is not a Federal one and if for instance I wanted to practice in Connecticut I would have to get a license from that State. If I practiced in Connecticut without a Connecticut physician's license I could and probably would go to jail for that.

The license to practice by a State once given, however, is unqualified in the sense that the State does not govern what each physician can or cannot do with their license and leaves it to the physician's individual judgment. The only limit on what the physician is allowed to do then is by the credentialing committee of the hospitals with which the doctor is affiliated. However when it comes to office based practice there is no such supervision giving rise to the situation where Board certified gynecologists are performing liposuction in their offices and otolaryngologists are performing breast implants in their offices. No matter how well intentioned these physicians, they often lack the training and experience to handle the complications that can arise from these procedures and hence the occasional scandal in the newspapers.

The best assurance for the patient considering liposuction, or in fact any cosmetic surgery, is to check the surgeon's background with the American Society of Plastic Surgeons (1-888- 4PLASTIC). If a physician you have enquired about is not a member of the Society they will simply say so and refuse any further questions about that doctor. Believe me however, they do not make mistakes and if they say that a surgeon you are interested is not a member then that surgeon is not a member!

The important thing about the surgeon who is certified by the American Board of Plastic Surgery is the fact that they have the necessary training, skills and background not only to perform your surgery but also to manage any complications that may arise during or after surgery. It is inevitable that any surgeon with a practice of any significance will have patients that develop infections, haematomas, wound problems, skin loss or even life-threatening emergencies.

In selecting a surgeon you should have the assurance that the surgeon you choose will have the abilities required to manage any such crisis because, ultimately, you are putting your life in that surgeons hands. The final benefit of selecting a surgeon, who is a member of the American Society of Plastic Surgeons is, that as a condition of membership in that Society, they have agreed to have their office operating rooms independently inspected and certified. This ensures that the operating room, where you will be operated meets the highest safety and hygiene standards. No other certification can give you that assurance.

# Chapter 12

## The Surgery Itself

Even for the patient who is well prepared through researching the subject the actual day of the surgery can be anxiety provoking. This is normal because, after all, this is surgery that you have chosen to undergo rather than something that was absolutely "medically" necessary. I can attest to these feelings having undergone liposuction myself.

On the day of surgery remember that you are to have nothing to eat or drink before going to the doctor's office apart from a sip of water to help swallow the pre-operative antibiotics or any other medications that your doctor has prescribed. At the office, you will meet the anesthesiologist responsible for your care during the surgery and you can discuss any particular concerns regarding the anesthesia with him or her, and then your surgeon will mark the areas to be worked on while you are in the standing position. (Remember everything changes when you lie down). Then, in the operating room, you will be given quite deep sedation to allow the surgeon to inject the areas to be worked on with the local anesthetic solution. My preference is to wait ten to fifteen minutes to allow the sedation to wear off and the local anesthetic to take full effect before I actually start the liposuction.

The benefit is that the patient is fully awake and can see the work being done as well as cooperate in moving their body to access difficult or hard to reach areas. If the patient prefers, instead, to be sedated throughout the procedure then we simply give the patient more sedation, but then the patient cannot cooperate by shifting positions during the surgery.

The liposuction, itself, usually takes about two hours and, after closing the incision sites the patient is placed in a compression garment. The purpose of this is to obliterate the potential space between the skin and underlying muscle where the fat used to be as well as helping the skin to shrink. The patient can usually leave for home shortly after the procedure is completed and because of the local anesthesia there is usually little pain at the sites worked on for three to four hours, but rather a numb feeling. This makes it relatively easy for the patient to return home, but they must be accompanied home by an adult, unless the procedure was done purely under local anesthesia.

Once home the patient should take the pain pills prescribed by their surgeon because once the local anesthesia wears off you can expect it to hurt and it is much better to have pain relief on board before the local anesthetic wears off. You may also experience some leakage of fluid from the incision sites. This is simply the excess local anesthetic fluid that was injected leaking out and nothing to worry about but it can be messy. In addition you will be swollen and probably black and blue. Over the next day or two it is important to get up and begin to move around even though there may be some discomfort as the muscles rub against the raw areas where the fat used to be. The patient is generally the best judge of when they can return to the activities of daily living but as a general rule if movement is bothersome then that is the body's way of telling you to rest just a little bit more and if it doesn't bother you then its okay to go ahead and do it.

I usually schedule the first post-operative visit for one week following the surgery at which time the stitches are removed. By this time, the swelling following surgery has begun to diminish and the outlines of the final result are becoming visible. The patient usually still has some black and blue bruises, but this also is dissipating. It is important at this visit to remind the patient that wearing a compression garment following surgery is important to help the skin shrink as the final result of liposuction is dependent on the skin shrinking evenly and smoothly over the fat that has been contoured.

Usually by the end of the first week all the patients are back to work, although many return to work by the third day. That's why Friday is the most popular day for liposuction because the patients want to be back to work by Monday! I like to see the patients again for follow-up at one month and three months after the surgery at which time post-operative pictures are taken to assess the results of surgery. By this time almost all the patients have forgotten what they looked like three months earlier and are quite amazed at the change in their appearance when I put the pre and post-op pictures side by side. Being able to fit into clothes that they had not worn for years or to go shopping for a new wardrobe is a delight for these patients and they usually come to the office decked out in their new finery.

This happy conclusion, however, is just the start of maintaining the patient's new body, and I usually take this opportunity to remind them of the inevitable truth, that if they take in calories in excess of what they burn off, they will store it as fat and they have to be vigilant in maintaining an exercise and diet program. Otherwise they may end up being one of the patients who say liposuction did not "work" for them.

*Remember, the end of the healing is simply the beginning of maintaining the new body that you have achieved.*

# Chapter 13

## Things you might want to discuss with your Surgeon

1) Ask about the surgeon's training, expertise and current affiliations. Don't be shy! You are planning to entrust your life to this person. Most surgeons will have some printed literature on themselves. Being a smart consumer however you should have already done your research on the surgeon before you even visit their office.

2) Take a tour of the operating room and recovery areas and ask about third party inspections of the operating facilities if they are in the Doctor's offices.

3) See before and after pictures of patients that the surgeon has actually operated on.

4) If you are seriously interested in surgery the surgeon may be able to arrange for you to speak to prior patients. I usually have former patients who have agreed to provide this service call the prospective patient.

5) Have any new techniques that I should know about been introduced since "Doctor, Is Liposuction Right for Me?" was published?

6) Write down here any other questions that have arisen in your mind while reading this book to ask during consultation.

# About the Author

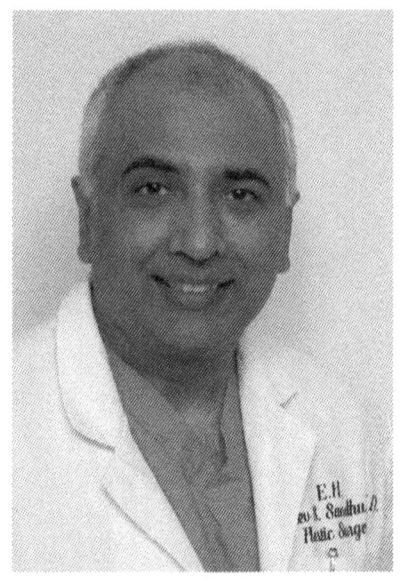

Baldev S. Sandhu M.D., is a Board Certified Plastic Surgeon and a member of the American Society of Plastic Surgeons.

Dr. Sandhu attended medical school at the University of Glasgow in Scotland and completed his training in Plastic and Reconstructive Surgery at Case Western Reserve University in 1988. Subsequently to that, he was the McDonald fellow in Pediatric Plastic Surgery at Akron Children's Hospital, and Assistant Professor of Plastic Surgery at the Medical College of Virginia.

He currently maintains a private practice in New York City and is working on his next book "The Plastic Surgeon's Diet Book".

www.ingramcontent.com/pod-product-compliance
Lightning Source LLC
Chambersburg PA
CBHW030845180526
45163CB00004B/1447